ANNIE PARKER CONFIDENTIAL

Live life beautifully ❀ by Shelli Pelly

28-DAY

California Sugar Cleanse

REBOOT YOUR LIFE!

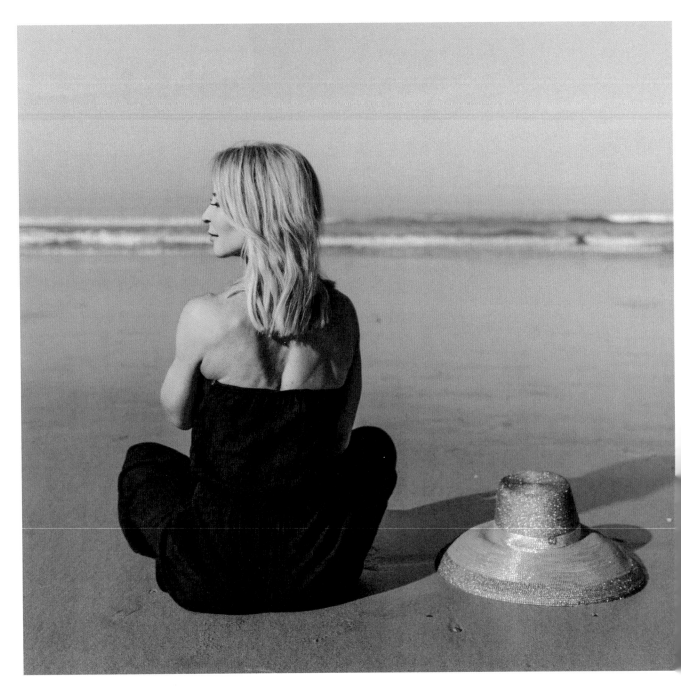

Annie Parker Confidential 28-Day California Sugar Cleanse

Cover Photo by Arielle Levy

Cover Design and Interior Typesetting and Layout by Melissa Williams Design

Published by Annie Parker Confidential by Shelli Pelly

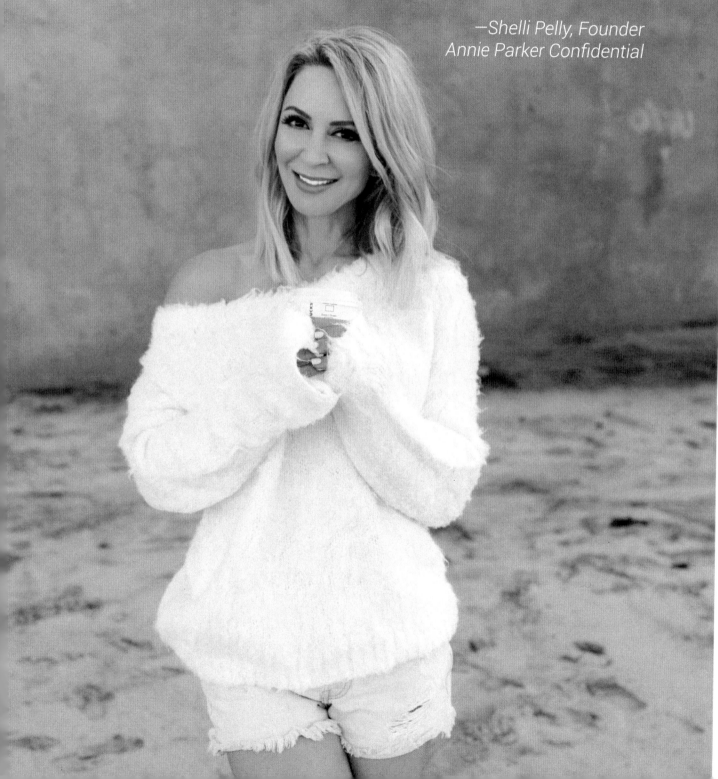

"My vision for APC is to create a community where women are safe, supported & accepted for exactly who they are, and encouraged to be everything they want to be."

—Shelli Pelly, Founder
Annie Parker Confidential

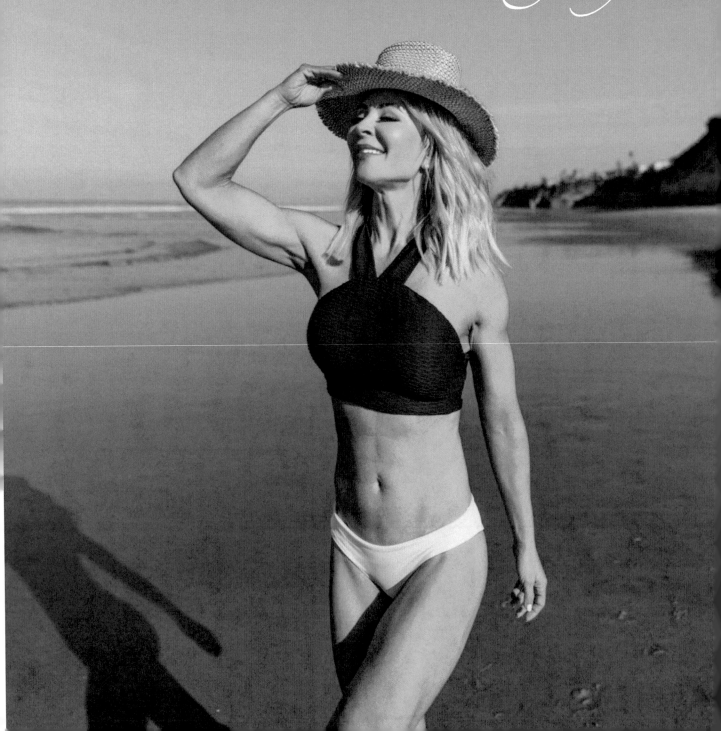

It's time to live
YOUR most amazing life!

Contents

WHY I WROTE THE 28-DAY CALIFORNIA SUGAR CLEANSE

My *Why* behind writing the 28-Day California Sugar Cleanse, is an extension of my Why behind starting the Annie Parker Confidential Blog & Brand: *A lifelong drive to build a platform from which I could help other women to become the very best, happiest, most joyful and fulfilled versions of themselves. Period.*

As a lifelong athlete & fitness fanatic, I have learned that the food we choose to put into our bodies lays the foundation upon which all else is built—or not. Food can nourish or it can destroy.

Knowing the importance of diet to our overall well-being, my objective was to create a do-able Sugar-Cleanse Program with healthy, easy to make no-sugar meals focused on whole & minimally processed foods. In the Cleanse you'll get 53 healthy meal & snack recipes made with lots of fresh veggies, fruits, whole grains, legumes, healthy fats—all with NO (added) SUGAR.

Why 28-Days

Ever heard the phrase "21-days to create a habit"? This hypothesis was actually brought about by a plastic surgeon in the 50's who started to note that it would take his patients about 21-days to get accustomed to seeing their new face & adjust to what was a new situation. In thinking about his own adjustment period to changes and new behaviors, he concluded that 21-days is the sweet-spot for an old habit or behavior to dissolve and for a new one to take root.

I chose 28-days to kick the sugar habit because . . . well, 21-days is 3 weeks and odd numbers bug me. It felt lopsided, if I'm being totally honest. Welcome to my all-the-labels-must-face-the-same-way, slightly OCD, Type-A world. Plus, I wanted to make damn sure that this new, healthier way of eating really took root!

4-weeks is long enough for the new behavior to take root, yet short enough for most to mentally Cowgirl-up during moments of weakness. Sort of like pushing through the last 30-seconds of a workout. When you know it's almost over—you'll hit the "X" button and drive through to the finish line.

Now of course I'm betting that once the 28-days are over, you will have gotten so accustomed to feeling and looking amazing—that going back to a sugar-filled diet won't be even remotely appealing.

We all learn from each other. As such, I welcome you into the APC community, where as women we connect, share, grow and learn in a positive, safe, fully supportive and friendship-based environment.

Enjoy discovering a healthier way of eating and by extension, a happier and more empowered way of living YOUR most amazing life!

Xoxo,

-Shelli

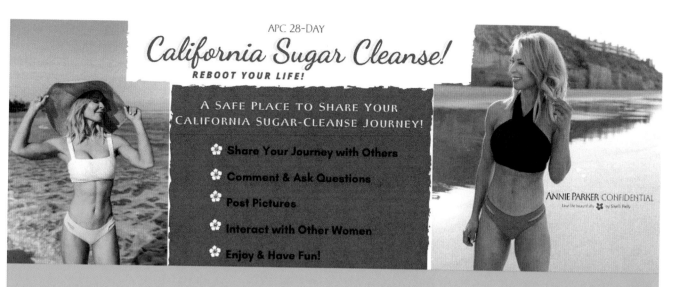

Want to join our Private APC 28-Day Sugar Cleanse Facebook Group?

This is a private group where we can all share our Sugar Cleanse journey! Only members can see posts and who's in the group. Here, you can:

✓ **Ask me questions & interact with other women!**

✓ **Share your successes—big & small!**

✓ **Post yummy meals you've made from the book**

✓ **Share new Recipes you love**

✓ **Get & give support from/to other women**

I've made this a safe, secure, supportive-only environment for women to share & encourage each other. My personal pet peeve are bullies, so I promise—no negativity will be allowed in our space. This is all about supporting, helping and celebrating each other. Join us—It's fun!

Join us! Click here: https://www.facebook.com/groups/APCSugarCleanse/

Or enter the link above into your browser. It'll take you directly to the page where you can click to join!

For Wellness + Beauty + Style + Fitness & Healthy Living— Connect with me everywhere!

Visit the Blog: www.AnnieParkerConfidential.com

30-Minute Workouts, Lite Recipes & more: @annieparkerconfidential

@annieparkerconfidential

@annieparkerconfidential

@annieparkerconfidential

Sugar

THE SILENT ASSASSIN

Sugar. It's sweet, delicious and it is toxic. Sort of like my first boyfriend.

It has silently, steadily woven its way into our entire food system like a cancer. First, in very obvious foods like cakes, cookies and ice creams—to less obvious products like spaghetti sauce, salad dressings and granola, all the way to *completely unexpected* products like protein bars, "healthy" bottled smoothies, low-fat foods, cereals and yogurts. It is everywhere—and it is killing us.

Sugar is marketed as sexy, attractive and exciting—think of how many times you've seen a celebrity pitching Coke, Pepsi or Sports drinks . . . all of which are *loaded* with added sugar. As in almost *double* a woman's *maximum* daily added-sugar allowance of 24-grams (more about this later) . . . *in one can of soda.* Insane.

Still, our beloved sugar is synonymous with love and celebration. Think of Valentine's Day, Birthdays, Special Occasions or holidays like Halloween, Easter, Christmas and Thanksgiving. I mean, it's *all* about the Benjamins. I mean the sugar, it's all about the sugar in one way or another.

Its Ubiquity Has Caused a Nation of Addicts

and some very wealthy food conglomerates

The problem is that sugar is no longer limited to just the obvious foods we've always known about. It's like a Silent Assassin, quietly, systematically working its way into our entire food system while strategically casting the spotlight on poor ole Fat and Carbs as the enemy to avoid. Ooooo! It's fat-free! Sound familiar? *Cough . . . Entenmann's . . . cough . . .*

The demonization of Fat & Carbs created 2 brand new trends in the marketspace: No/Low-Fat and No/Low-Carb. In turn, these trends spawned new and highly lucrative bandwagon-opportunities for food manufacturers. How?

Well, Sales 101 says:

Start with an old product (cheaper & easier than starting from scratch)— tweak it a little, then market the bejeezus out of it as something new, sexy and exciting that people <u>must have.</u> We used to call it "Sell the sizzle, not the steak."

8

ANNIE PARKER CONFIDENTIAL
Live life beautifully ❁ by Shelli Pelly

In the case of a food manufacturer, they could simply dip into their existing product line, and make non-fat, low-fat, low-carb and no-carb versions of any given product in order to capitalize on the trends and . . . Bingo! Sales gold. Unfortunately, when you take fat or carbs *out* of a food, it tastes like cardboard. To make it taste good—and ergo "sellable" to the consumer, *they add Sugar!*

And therein lies the problem. Sugar is highly addicting. The more we eat, the more we crave and want it. It changes our taste buds such that foods lacking the sweetness to which we've grown accustomed, don't taste very good. So, guess what happens? Yup. Food gets a sugar bump to meet our taste demands. It's a vicious cycle—and with this Program, we're going to jump off the sugar merry-go-round and into a healthier, happier lane.

Knowing Your "Why"

Before we jump into the Program and start talking *solutions*, I want you to truly reflect upon *your* Why. Why did you pick up this book? *Why* are you interested in clearing sugar from your life? *What* motivates you? *What* do you want from this?

Reflecting upon your "why" will define your *focus* and your *intention,* which in turn provides clarity and a rudder guiding you to your goal. It'll be that kick-in-the-pants that says, "keep going," when things get challenging or you're tempted to revert back to what's known and comfortable. *Envision what you want—and don't take your eye off the prize.*

My Why . . . Why I Wrote the Program

My *Why* behind writing the Program is an extension of my *Why* behind starting Annie Parker Confidential: A lifelong drive *(sometimes it feels more like an overwhelming "pull")* to build a platform from which I could help other women to become the very best, happiest, joyful and most fulfilled versions

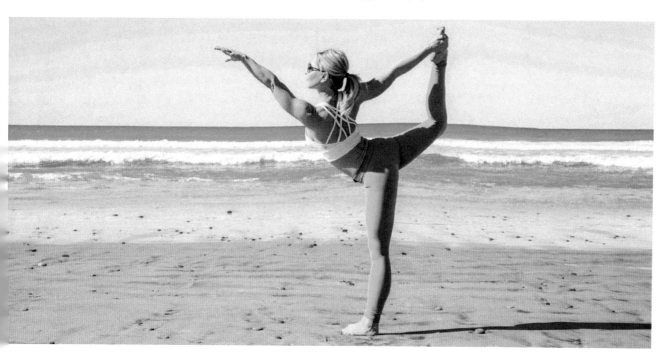

of themselves. We all learn from each other. I wanted to create a platform—a community where as women, we could all connect, share, grow and learn in a positive, safe, fully supportive and friendship-based environment.

Knowing the importance that our diet plays in our overall well-being, I wanted to create a doable Program, for a targeted period of time, that would help women discover a healthier way of eating and by extension, a happier and more empowered way of living.

The Deal with our Diet

The food we put into our bodies is the *foundation* upon which all else is built—or not. Food can nourish *or* destroy.

For better or worse, the food we choose to ingest affects our:

✓ **Insides**

✓ **Physical health**

✓ **Energy level**

✓ **Moods and by extension the way we treat others**

✓ **Mind clarity and acuity**

✓ **Desire to fully engage in the world and our overall well-being**

✓ **It affects our weight, our skin, hair and the quality with which we age.**

One of the biggest offenders and threats to all of the above is *too much added-Sugar* in our diets. It may sound somewhat hyperbolic at first (that's what I thought), but it's not. It is *incredibly harmful* to us and for that reason, I share with you Best Practices on what I've learned about the harmful effects of Sugar, through a combination of research, my personal "no-sugar" practice, and a lifetime of fitness and healthy eating.

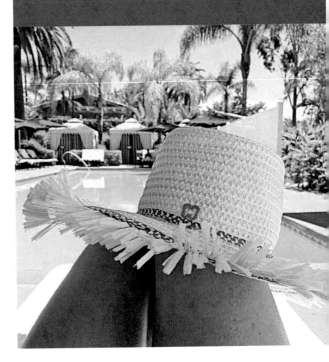

Safety first . . .

To be clear, I am not a Licensed Nutritionist *and* the Program isn't intended to be a substitute for medical advice or guidance from a healthcare professional. Before starting on any new diet, eating program or fitness journey you should *always* consult with a medical professional first. The Recipes provided in the Program are not geared towards any specific dietary needs, dietary restrictions or allergies so please just use common sense!

ANNIE PARKER CONFIDENTIAL
Live life beautifully ❀ by Shelli Pelly

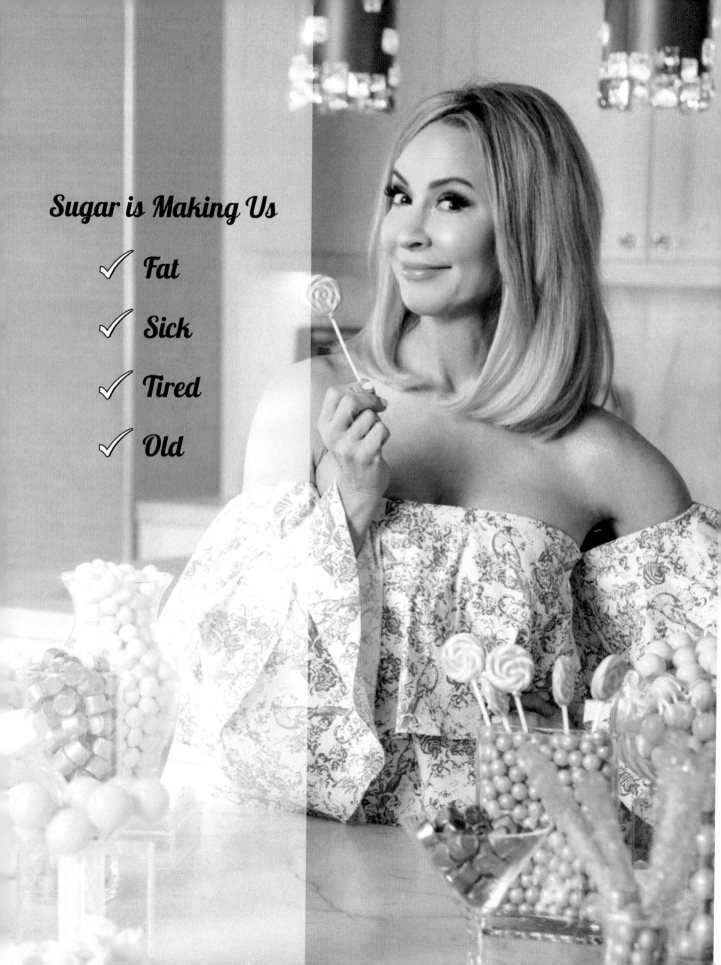

Sugar is Making Us

✓ Fat

✓ Sick

✓ Tired

✓ Old

Sugar is Making Us . . .

FAT, SICK, TIRED, OLD & DEPRESSED ADDICTS

I know. I'm just fun-in-a-bucket. But seriously—let's first understand the issue, then take actionable steps to stop doing that which harms us. Sugar is making us fat, sick, tired, old and depressed.

It is ruining our skin, accelerating the aging process, clouding our brains, and playing a key role in keeping us from being everything we are meant to be.

The ubiquity of *added*-sugar in our foods *(not the naturally occurring sugars in whole fruits, veggies or dairy products)* has created a nation of Sugar Addicts.

Sound like an embellishment? What would you call a person who knowingly puts toxic substances into their body, because they *need* the feeling or high that substance provides? They know it's killing them, yet the feeling, the high is all they can see. We'd call that person an addict.

Sugar is as Addicting as Cocaine

Ever notice that once you start on a bag of cookies it's super hard to stop? Or the more sugar you eat—the more you crave? It's not you or your willpower. It's the sugar, sugar. I mean, I'm a fan of personal responsibility—but let's be fair to ourselves . . .

Sugar is addicting—and that's not hyperbole. *The research actually says that our brains cannot tell the difference between sugar and cocaine.* That's why we sometimes get that panicky NEED for something sweet and the feeling does not go away until you feed it. Been there. Many times.

4 Reasons to Stop Eating Sugar

1. It Makes Us Fat

Sugar is void of nutrients, vitamins and fiber which means you are eating airy, empty calories and never feeling full. That's why you can eat an entire bag of cookies and still feel hungry. Guess what happens next? Yup. We reach for more food in an effort to feel sated, resulting in eating more and more calories.

Add-in the fact that Sugar is extremely addicting—causing hardcore cravings, and you've got a vicious cycle. Eat—crave—eat—crave—eat . . .

But it's not only the additional calories we're eating—it's the INSULIN SURGE that sugar causes in our body—which promotes weight gain.

Insulin Surge says: "Stop burning fat, Start storing it."

Inside of our bodies, our pancreas creates a hormone called insulin. Insulin is released into the bloodstream to help regulate our blood sugar by transferring said blood sugar

ANNIE PARKER CONFIDENTIAL
Live life beautifully 🌸 by Shelli Pelly

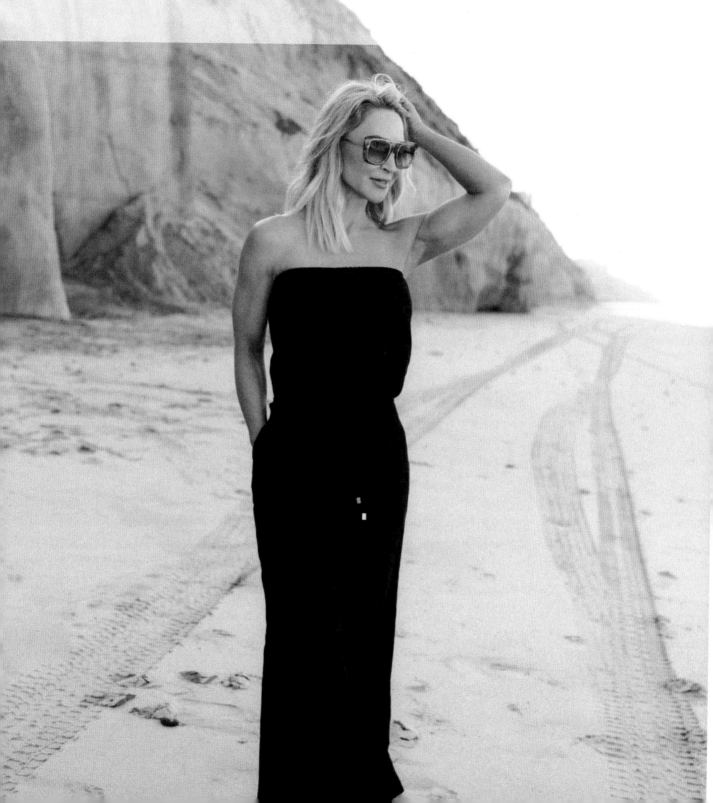

"It's not just the calories, it's the way sugar interacts with our insides, signaling the body to STORE fat, not BURN it."

into our bloodstream and into our cells. In other words, it keeps everything running smoothly and systematically. When we eat foods with too much sugar, our pancreas goes into overdrive to produce enough insulin to accommodate the rush of sugar we've just ingested.

This is called an *Insulin Surge*. Think of it like the difference between a light sprinkle of rain, and a torrential downpour. Too much sugar = torrential downpour and the pancreas is trying desperately to put out enough rain buckets to keep from drowning.

This insulin surge says to our body:

"Hey, there's plenty of energy available so I need you to stop burning fat and start storing it."

This why we gain or cannot lose weight, eating a high-sugar diet. It's not just the extra calories—it is the way in which too much sugar interacts with our insides, causing an insulin surge which tells the body to store fat—not burn it.

2. It Makes Us Sick

Too much Sugar can also have some serious health consequences, including:

✓ **Diabetes**

✓ **Stroke**

✓ **Suppression of the immune system**

✓ **Obesity related deaths**

✓ **High blood pressure**

3. It Makes Us Lethargic, Depressed, and Moody

If you've never had a sugar-high, followed by a sugar-crash . . . You probably aren't reading this! Sugar crashes are the worst. I eat a pretty healthy diet, but admittedly I have always had a huge sweet tooth that I'd indulge every once in a while. The carrot cake, cheesecake or buttercream cupcakes were so stinking good going down—but shortly thereafter, it was time to "pay the piper."

I'd start to get *super* grumpy, irritable, restless and snappy. Next I'd start feeling

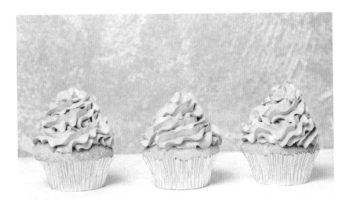

moody, down & depressed which is out of character. Of course, this was the sugar crash. Despite these effects—no joke, I'd finish off any remaining cupcakes . . . THAT is the addiction!!!

4. It Ruins and Ages Our Skin

All of the expensive creams and skin lasers are a waste of money, if you're still eating a high-sugar diet. While there are other factors that contribute to premature or accelerated aging of the skin, such as sun, stress, poor diet and smoking—Sugar is by far the worst offender.

ANNIE PARKER CONFIDENTIAL
Live life beautifully ❀ by Shelli Pelly

3 Ways Sugar Damages Our Skin

1. Sugar Damages Collagen and Elastin

Collagen is the protein that "plumps" our skin giving it a fresh, youthful look while Elastin (just think of "elastic") is what allows our skin to snap-back into place after we smile, frown or make a funny face. When we eat a high-sugar diet, it causes the collagen and elastin to become more brittle, and stiff. Consequently, our skin breaks down and looks thinner and wrinkly.

Too much sugar also creates more testosterone, which enlarges our pores & stimulates oil production. The result? A rougher, ruddier complexion. Like a guy . . . Yeah, no bueno.

It *also* becomes more prone to environmental and UV ray damage . . . yeah. That's not a good thing.

2. Sugar is dehydrating

Sugar is a dehydrating agent, which causes increased oil production in our skin. In addition, sugar affects water binding—which is why our skin can look less oxygenated and dull. Instead, skin takes on a lackluster, sallow appearance with dark under-eye circles.

3. Sugar is an inflammatory

Yup—it's good ole' inflammation again. Because Sugar is an inflammatory food, it causes inflammation within our body. When we eat high-sugar foods like baked goods, soda, flavored yogurts, most bottled smoothies (yes!)—they go directly into our gut for processing, then into our bloodstream causing our insulin to spike.

This insulin spike subsequently increases the inflammation in our skin which can aggravate skin conditions like psoriasis, rosacea, eczema and result in acne flare-ups. It also increases inflammation in our body, which breaks down collagen and elastin, resulting in sagging skin and wrinkles.

In short, your body is reacting in spades—to something that it knows is harmful. Listen to it!

Specifics Please!!
How Much Sugar is OK?

I know—we need specifics, people!! I got-cha. Here's the deal . . .

According to the Diabetes Council, Americans by far have the *highest* daily average of added-sugar intake at *126-grams per person!* The *maximum* daily sugar intake for women should be no more than *24-grams* or *6-teaspoons*. For men, no more than *36-grams* or *9*-teaspoons. This, according to the American Diabetes Council. This means that on average, we are consuming 4–5x the maximum recommendation. That's insane.

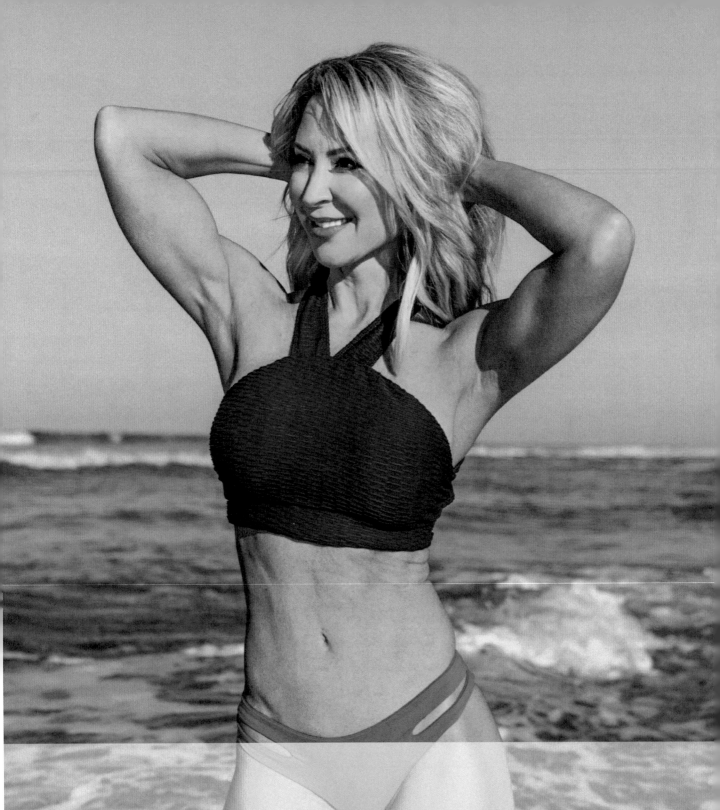

"Sugar damages collagen & elastin, causing skin to break down and look thinner and wrinkly."

1 cup, Grape Nuts Cereal = 10 grams sugar

1 cup, Low-Fat Vanilla Yogurt, Yoplait = 29 grams sugar

8-oz Fresh Squeezed Orange Juice = 20 grams sugar

Total = 59 grams of Sugar

Crazy right? 59-grams of sugar for breakfast and we've still got the rest of the day. That's 2.5x more than our total daily allowance. In one meal.

HERE'S A BETTER ALTERNATIVE:

Steel Cut Oats, fresh blueberries, unsweetened almond milk, chopped walnuts

Coffee with favorite nut-milk

= 0 grams added sugar

Far from feeling deprived, you'll find the alternative version so much more satisfying. It will leave you feeling sated and energetic, with stable blood sugar and clarity of mind. *Sugar-free* is not about sacrifice and deprivation, to the contrary. It's about clearing away the cobwebs of sugar-addiction including lethargy, inflammation, too much weight, mind-fog and moodiness to a life where you look and feel more vibrant, energetic, and happier. It's just a matter of understanding healthier options, which is exactly what this Program offers.

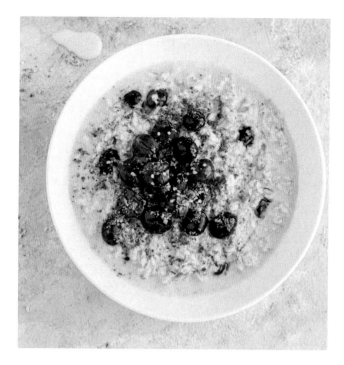

No-Sugar vs. Low-Sugar

Choosing your lane after the 28-day Program

The focus of the 28-Day Sugar Cleanse—Reboot Your Life! is simple:

Eliminate all added sugar for 28-days and reboot your life.

Don't worry—it's actually not that hard and I promise you won't suffer . . . that much. Kidding—you'll be fine.

After the 28-days, it's your decision whether to stick to a *No-Sugar Lifestyle* or opt for a *Low-Sugar Lifestyle*. The *No-Sugar Lifestyle* is just a continuation of the 28-Day Program, which is no-added sugars but does allow for the *naturally occurring sugars* found in whole fruits, some veggies and dairy.

A *Low-Sugar Lifestyle* is staying under 24-grams of added sugar per day (women), under 36-grams for men. Of course this assumes approval by a medical professional, especially if you have underlying health concerns.

Personally...

Personally, I'm very close to No-Sugar, but if something gets by me—I don't want to be a hypocrite, so I say "I'm Low-Sugar." That being said, I *do* stay well below 24-grams just by virtue of the foods we buy (all in the Program!). On average, I probably have anywhere from 0–5 grams of added-sugar per day. I'm fine with that.

It's just about feeling healthy, energetic and engaged. There's only one YOU! Don't deprive the world of your light.

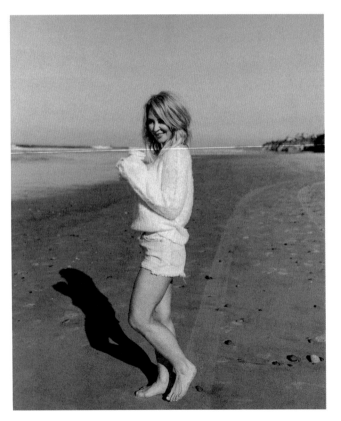

Added-Sugar vs Natural Occurring Sugars

Why do I keep saying *added*-sugar, and not just *sugar?* Good question. Most of us think of "sugar" as the unhealthy kind, but sugar is also found in whole fruits, some veggies and dairy. These sugars are referred to as *naturally occurring sugars* because they . . . ummm . . . occur NATURALLY and aren't added. So, we use the terms "added" and "naturally recurring" to make the distinction.

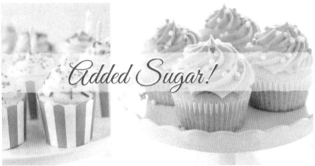

Added-Sugars are the unhealthy, refined sugars that are added to foods during processing to make them taste better, add texture, shelf-life and/or drive down the price.

They're most always found in processed, packaged foods, candy, ice cream, baked goods and even in many foods labeled healthy, like flavored yogurts, bottled smoothies, many low-fat or non-fat foods. Oh, and of course most restaurant food.

ANNIE PARKER CONFIDENTIAL
Live life beautifully ❀ by Shelli Pelly

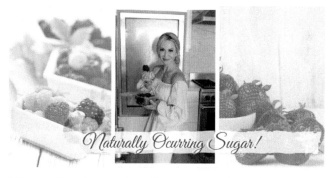
Naturally Occurring Sugar!

Naturally Occurring Sugars are found in foods like *whole* fruits, vegetables or dairy products—and do not cause the insulin surge or harmful effects that added-sugars do. Because of this, naturally occurring sugars *do not count* towards the 24-gram daily allowance of a Low-Sugar diet. Notice that I said *whole* fruits.

Whole Fruit vs Fruit Juice

Just say "no" to da juice!

Fruit contains fructose, which is a *naturally occurring sugar* found in all fruits. When eating the *whole* fruit, fructose does *not* have the harmful effects that added-sugars do. This is because the fiber in the whole fruit is intact and the sugar is contained within its cells. Since it takes our digestive system a while to break-down these cells, fructose is released into our bloodstream slowly—avoiding the dreaded Insulin Spike (sugar rush).

Fruit juices (*yes, even 100% fresh squeezed or pressed*) are a NO. Why? Because essentially a glass of juice is created by separating out the fiber, leaving you with a glass of sugar and carbs. With the fiber removed, the fructose is absorbed into your system super fast, causing an Insulin Spike (sugar rush).

Shades of a "No-Sugar" Lifestyle

People define a "No-Sugar Lifestyle" in varying degrees. For example, some believe this means no sugar of *any kind*, including those in whole fruits, some veggies and dairy.

Others (including the American Diabetes Association) do not count the natural sugars of whole fruits, towards the recommended 24-gram daily maximum, and therefore include whole fruits as part of their lifestyle. I fall into this category.

Personally, I have a hard time believing that a whole, natural piece of fruit should be banned from a healthy lifestyle, so I include it in my daily diet. In the end, it's your call on which feels best to you. You're the boss of you!

6 "Healthy Foods" That Can Be Sugar-Bombs!

Watch for hidden sugars in these foods

1. Yogurt

Yogurt has always been thought of as a healthy choice, but nowadays finding one *without* added sugar is the exception rather than the other way around. Pretty much any flavored yogurt is going to have Added Sugar—including "Low-Fat" versions. Check it out for yourself next time you're in the grocery store.

Light & Fit Vanilla Greek Yogurt—7-grams of sugar. Yoplait Light Harvest Peach—10-grams. That's almost *half* of a woman's maximum daily sugar allowance of 24-gram. In one little tiny yogurt container. Better option: Choose Plain Unsweetened Greek Yogurt and add your own fresh fruit and chopped nuts. Way healthier.

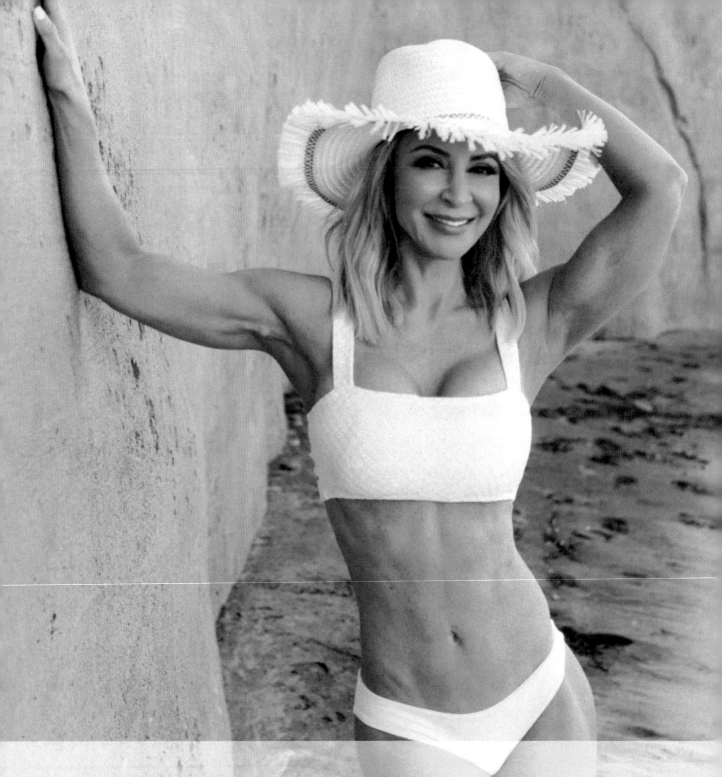

6 "Healthy Foods" That Can Be Sugar-Bombs!

2. Granola

Flat out, most Granola is very high in sugar and calories for a very small portion. The main ingredient—oats, are healthy in and of themselves but when combined with honey or syrup plus a number of other sweeteners, the sugar & calories are off the chart.

KIND Honey & Oat Granola snack has 11-grams of sugar in only 2/3 a cup! Granola is delicious and addicting once the bag is opened . . . or so I've heard, haha. Never have I ever . . . had only 2/3 a cup, so you know—just a heads up.

3. Spaghetti Sauce

Yup. That's the scary thing about how far off-track our food-system has gotten. It's no longer just the usual cake & cookie suspects. Added sugars are often hidden in foods we'd never suspect—like spaghetti sauce or ketchup. To be fair, spaghetti sauce will contain some natural sugar from the tomatoes, but many also have added sugar.

Either make your own, or just double check the Ingredients and see if sugar of any form is listed.

4. Protein Bars

Protein. The minute we see or hear "protein" most people automatically assume it must be healthy. Eating foods high in Protein is a great way to feel full and sated, which is why Protein bars have become so popular. The issue is that many bars have slowly evolved into bars of sugar with protein added. I'm exaggerating, but you get my point.

Some have well over 20-grams of added-sugar!! Knowledge is power—flip the bar over and Read the label (I'll show you exactly how, in the next section!). It's always better to have actual real, whole food for a snack—like an apple and nut butter, or any of the Sugar-Free snacks in the Program. In a pinch, just make sure you choose bars with no added-sugar.

5. Sports drinks, Vitamin Water, Bottled Smoothies, Iced Tea, Fancy Coffees, Sodas

I know. Bummer, right? The truth is, one of *the easiest* and best things you can do for your body—is to simply drink water when you're thirsty. Sports drinks, Vitamin Water, Bottled smoothies, fancy coffee drinks are most always FULL of sugar and empty calories. Water is Queen, *and* she's good for your pretty skin! Happy face.

6. Ketchup

Obvious to some, not to others. Condiments are foods that we sometimes don't think much of, but ketchup is *full* of sugar. Sad face. So, not only will the burger and fries get 'cha—so will the flipping ketchup. Just ONE measly tablespoon of Heinz ketchup has a full teaspoon of ketchup which equates to 4 grams of sugar. That's 4 grams—in the daily 24 gram max the ADA sets for women. No!

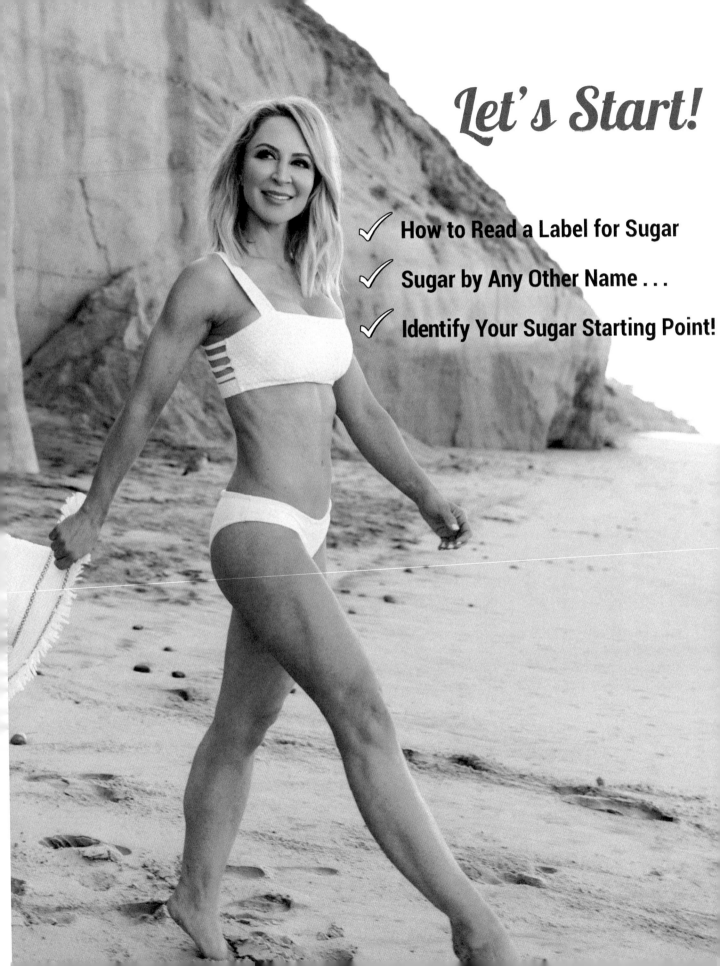

Let's Start!

✓ **How to Read a Label for Sugar**

✓ **Sugar by Any Other Name . . .**

✓ **Identify Your Sugar Starting Point!**

How to Read a Label for Sugar

DO THESE THINGS BEFORE IT GOES IN YOUR CART!

A few quick things to know about identifying "Sugar" on labels. First, we are looking to avoid ADDED Sugar—but how do you tell? There are 3 quick ways:

1. Some products have a separate line item that says "Added Sugars"—which makes it super easy. ***See Example #1, KIND BAR.***

2. Other products do not have a separate line item. They just lump Natural & Added together in one line-item labeled "Sugars," so we cannot automatically tell if the sugar grams are Naturally Occurring or Added. The good news is that this is temporary. Here's why:

   Effective January 1, 2021—the FDA (Food & Drug Administration) has mandated that all food manufacturers must have a separate line-item for Added Sugar (like our Kind Bar example). That'll make it way easier for us! Today, some manufacturers have implemented the changes, others have not.

   For now—a quick scan of the Ingredients Label will tell you if there are Added Sugars. (*See the following list of Other Common Names for Sugar*). See Example #2, OR-GANIC MARINARA SAUCE.

3. If I do not see any form of Sugar on the Ingredients label—I know the Sugar grams are Naturally Occurring and are OK to eat. ***See Example #3, CHOBANI PLAIN GREEK YOGURT***

KIND BAR

On the label, I see: *"Total Sugars 5g."* Underneath, it says *"Incl. 4g of Added Sugars"*. That's really all I need to know. It has Added-Sugar, so I put it back. By default the other gram of sugar is probably a naturally occurring sugar in some of the nuts.

ORGANIC MARINARA SAUCE

On the label, I see *Sugars 4g*. There isn't a separate line-item for Added-Sugars. A quick scan of the Ingredients and I see "Organic Sugar"—which, is added-sugar, so back it goes. Oh—also, if you choose a Low-Sugar Lifestyle after the Program, be sure to look at the Serving Size. They're almost always super small. Here, the serving size is ½ a cup. Most people will have more than that—so you'll want to factor that in.

DARK CHOCOLATE NUTS & SEA SALT

Nutrition Facts	Amount/Serving	% Daily Value	Amount/Serving	% Daily Value
	Total Fat 15g	**19%**	**Total Carb.** 16g	**6%**
	Sat. Fat 3g	**15%**	Fiber 7g	**25%**
Serving size 1 bar (40g)	*Trans* Fat 0g		Total Sugars 5g	
	Polyunsaturated Fat 3.5g		Incl. 4g of Added Sugars	**8%**
	Monounsaturated Fat 8g		Sugar Alcohol 0g	
Calories per serving 200	**Cholesterol** 0mg	**0%**	**Protein** 6g	
	Sodium 140mg	**6%**		
	Vitamin D 0% • Calcium 4% • Iron 6% • Potassium 4%			

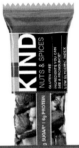

INGREDIENTS: Almonds, peanuts, chicory root fiber, honey, palm kernel oil, sugar, glucose syrup, rice flour, unsweetened chocolate, cocoa powder, sea salt, soy lecithin, natural flavor, cocoa butter.

Allergen Information: Contains almonds, peanuts and soy.

Made in a facility that processes tree nuts and sesame seeds.

May contain nut shell fragments.

Nutrition Facts

Serving Size 1/2 cup (113g)
Servings Per Container about 6

Amount Per Serving

Calories 45 | Calories from Fat 10

	% Daily Value*
Total Fat 1g	**1%**
Saturated Fat 0g	**0%**
Trans Fat 0g	
Cholesterol 0mg	**0%**
Sodium 480mg	**20%**
Total Carbohydrate 8g	**3%**
Dietary Fiber 2g	**8%**
Sugars 4g	
Protein 2g	
Vitamin A 6% • Vitamin C 15%	
Calcium 6% • Iron 6%	

*Percent Daily Values are based on a 2,000 calorie diet. Your daily values may be higher or lower depending on your calorie needs:

	Calories:	2,000	2,500
Total Fat	Less than	65g	80g
Sat Fat	Less than	20g	25g
Cholesterol	Less than	300mg	300mg
Sodium	Less than	2,400mg	2,400mg
Total Carbohydrate		300g	375g
Dietary Fiber		25g	30g

Calories per gram:
Fat 9 • Carbohydrate 4 • Protein 4

INGREDIENTS: ORGANIC TOMATO PUREE, ORGANIC TOMATOES, SALT, ORGANIC ONIONS, ORGANIC SOYBEAN OIL, ORGANIC SUGAR, ORGANIC PARMESAN CHEESE (CULTURED PASTEURIZED ORGANIC MILK, SALT, POWDERED CELLULOSE, MICROBIAL ENZYMES), ORGANIC GARLIC POWDER, ORGANIC GARLIC, ORGANIC BASIL, ORGANIC OREGANO.

CONTAINS: MILK

CERTIFIED ORGANIC

CERTIFIED ORGANIC BY
QUALITY ASSURANCE INTERNATIONAL

CHOBANI PLAIN YOGURT

On the label, I see *Sugars 6g*. A quick scan of the Ingredients and I do *not* see any form of Sugar. That means the Sugar content is just Naturally Occurring. This goes into my cart!

Serving Size: 1 cup
Serving Per Container: 4
Amount Per Serving

Calories: 120

	% Daily Value*
Calcium	25%
Cholest. 10mg	3%
Dietary Fiber 0g	0%
Fat Cal. 0Cal	
Iron	0%
Potassium 320mg	10%
Protein 22g	44%
Sat. Fat 0g	0%
Sodium 85mg	4%
Sugars 6g	
Total Carb. 9g	3%
Total Fat 0g	0%
Trans Fat 0g	
Vitamin A	0%
Vitamin C	0%

1. First I look at the Sugar grams.

2. Next, to confirm that the "sugar" is Naturally Recurring - not Added, I look at the Ingredients.

3. I don't see any sugars listed in the Ingredients, so this is GOOD! Confirms that the sugars are Natural. This is a good product to eat!

* Percentage of Daily Values are based on a 2,000 calorie diet.

Ingredients:
Nonfat Yogurt (Cultured Pasteurized Nonfat Milk).

Heads-up, the front of the package is for marketing. I call this "The Spin." It may say something like Low-fat, Organic, Healthy, Nutritious, Low-sugar, etc. This is where the food company entices you to buy the product by making it appear (right or wrong), that it's a healthy choice. Take it with a grain of salt, then flip the package over and read the Label for the real 411!

The First 3-Ingredients Matter

Ingredients are listed beginning with *the most prevalent ingredient first*, ending with least prevalent. So, the first 3 are going to make up the majority of the product. Do you see sugar (or any form like—glucose, fructose, sucrose, syrup of any kind) in the first 3? Probably not a healthy choice.

Knowledge is power. As you're grocery shopping and deciding whether to place something in your cart—Stop, Drop and Roll: Read the label. Know what you're buying.

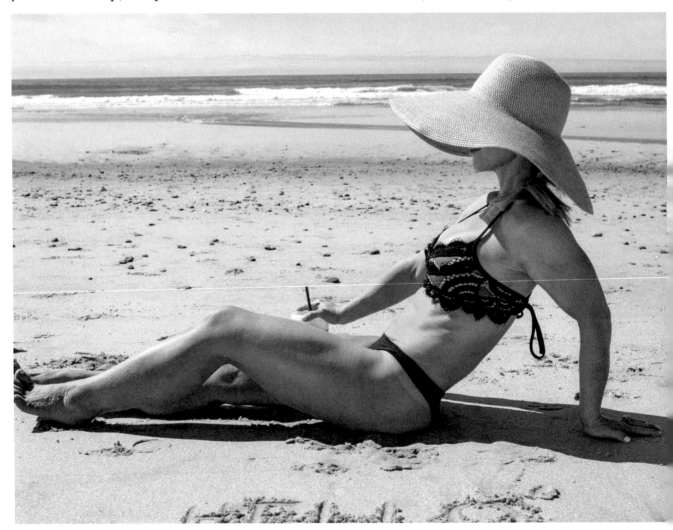

ANNIE PARKER CONFIDENTIAL
Live life beautifully ❀ by Shelli Pelly

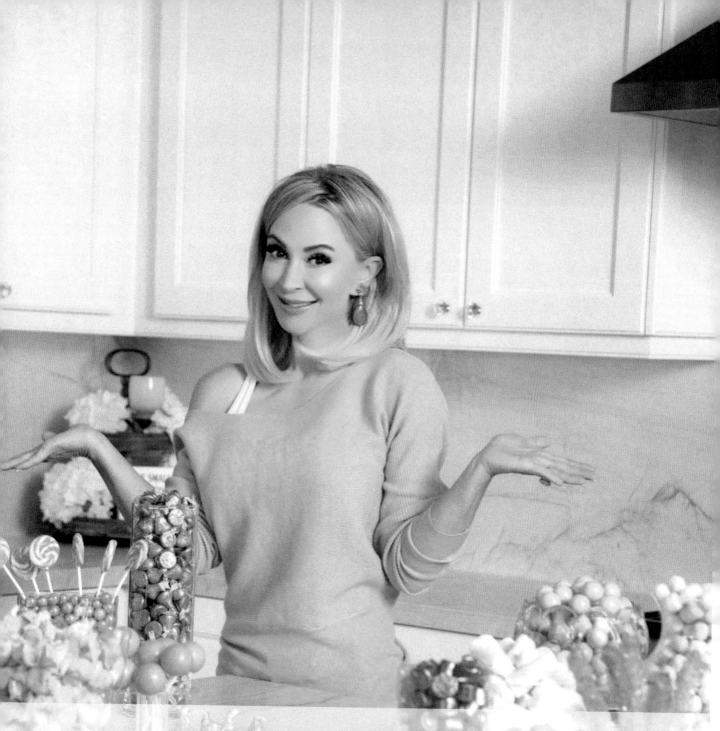

Sugar by Any Other Name is Still . . . Sugar

Watch Out for These Most Common Names for Sugar

Sugar By Any Other Name . . .

WATCH OUT FOR THESE MOST COMMON NAMES FOR SUGAR

Food labels are sneaky little bastards, especially when it comes to playing hide-the-sugar. There are so many different names for different types of sugar, it's mind boggling. Read labels carefully. Here are some of the most common names for sugar to watch-out for:

1. Sugar, aka Sucrose and *anything* containing the word "Sugar" in it
   (*beet sugar, brown sugar, cane sugar, organic sugar, raw sugar, date sugar, etc*).

2. High-Fructose Corn Syrup, *anything* containing the word "Syrup" in it
   (*Carob syrup, maple syrup, Buttered syrup*)

3. Glucose

4. Fructose

5. Honey

6. Fruit Juice

7. Fruit Juice from Concentrate

8. Barley Malt

9. Treacle

10. Dextrose

11. Dextrin

12. Maltrose

13. Muscovado

14. Mannose

14. Molasses or Blackstrap molasses

15. Panocha

16. Cane juice crystals

17. Caramel

18. Evaporated cane juice

19. Florida crystals

20. Sweet Sorghum

21. Sucanat

ANNIE PARKER CONFIDENTIAL
Live life beautifully ❀ by Shelli Pelly

Identify Your Sugar Starting Point!

How much sugar are you eating each day, on average? Would you guess it's under 24-grams, under 50-grams? Higher? Let's get a gauge on it. Don't stress—knowledge is power and you've got to know where you are, to get where you're going.

Here's What to Do:

1. *Go into your pantry.* Select foods you'd typically eat in any given day. Turn the package or can over, and simply jot down how many grams of sugar per serving in that item.

2. *Make sure to read the serving size.* They're usually super small, and most of us will naturally have at least 2-servings! That means we're eating even more sugar than we think.

   For example, my ex-favorite pasta sauce has 4-grams of sugar for a 1/2-cup serving. When measuring out my typical serving, I found that I'd usually have 1-cup which is 2-servings according to the label. That meant I was eating 8-grams of sugar . . . just in a little "healthy" marinara sauce. Not good. I changed brands.

3. *Be sure to include drinks!* Things like Sports drinks, Vitamin Waters, and Specialty Coffee drinks can have loads of sugar in them. Be sure to include those in your analysis.

4. *Add it all up.* Are you generally under 24-grams per day, or over? By how much? Either way—you've got a starting point.

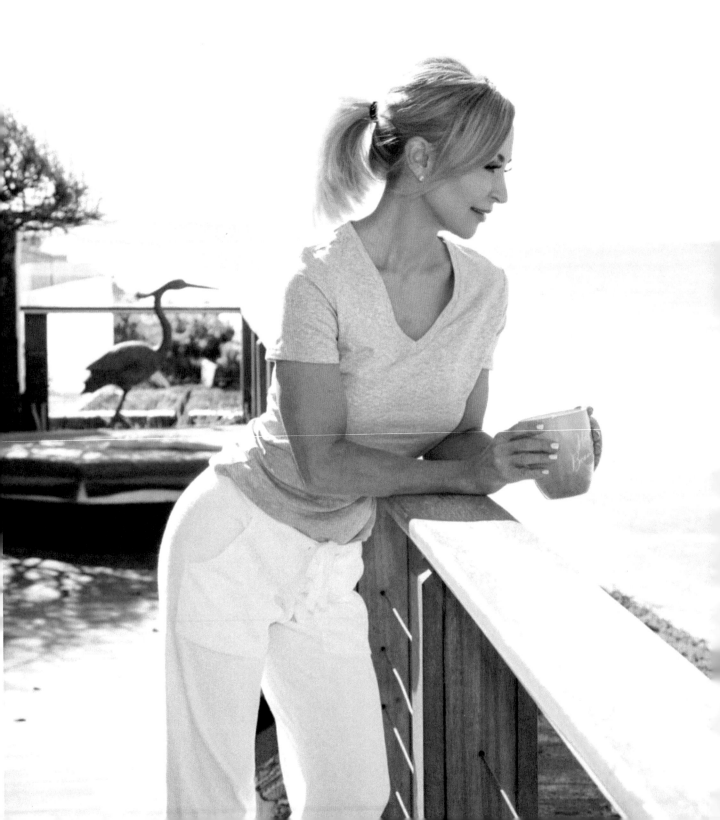

"You're never too old and it's never too late to begin living YOUR most amazing life!

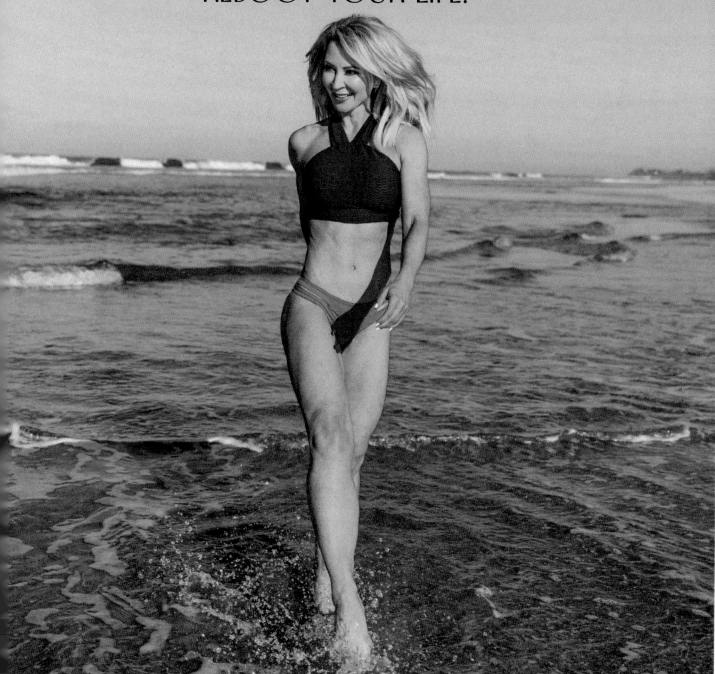

ANNIE PARKER CONFIDENTIAL

Live life beautifully by Shelli Pelly

28-DAY

California Sugar Cleanse

REBOOT YOUR LIFE!

28-Day California Sugar Cleanse

WHAT IT IS

The **28-Day California Sugar Cleanse—Reboot Your Life!** is a Program filled with healthy, wholesome, *No-Added-Sugar* Meals and Recipes designed to free your system from the negative effects of sugar addiction and *Reboot Your Life* onto a healthier, happier, joy-filled path!

Enjoy choosing from a variety of deliciously healthy Breakfast, Lunch, Dinner and Snacks recipes with Whole and/or *Minimally* Processed foods, *all with no added-sugars.*

This is an introduction to a healthier, happier way of eating. One that you will actually *want* to adopt for a lifetime because of the amazing way it will make you look, feel and think!

You won't want to eat sugary crap after doing this Program.

5 Reasons You'll Love It:

1. Easy & Delicious

All of the meal ideas and recipes are yummy, healthy and easy to make. I use a lot of fresh vegetables, whole fruits, whole grains, lean meat and fresh seafoods so you'll feel vibrant, healthy and amazing!

2. A Focus on Nutritious Whole Foods, not Highly-Processed

My vision for APC has always been about empowering women to *"Live Your Most Amazing Life!"* A large part of that is evolving and learning smart ways to enjoy a healthy, clean lifestyle. One that energizes and propels you forward.

Highly-processed foods are not a part of a healthy lifestyle and are therefore avoided in the Program—that includes those labeled sugar-free. Why? Because "no-sugar" packaged products with an ingredient list 3-inches long, filled with words we can barely pronounce aren't nourishing for our bodies, sugar or no-sugar.

At APC, it's all about nourishing our bodies with *whole and minimally processed foods, with limited ingredients and no-added sugars.* We're going to focus on preparing easy, healthy meals that nourish and fuel our bodies in addition to ridding it of sugar.

3. Flexibility

You're *not* restricted to the meals in the program. These meals are simply my personal favorites that I wanted to share, to help make your journey easier and more enjoyable. Think of them as "how-to" examples and inspiration for your own creations, as you learn how to eat Sugar-Free for life.

ANNIE PARKER CONFIDENTIAL
Live life beautifully ❀ by Shelli Pelly

4. Skin & Body Love

You'll love the positive differences in the quality of your skin, waistline, energy and mindset 2-3 weeks into the Program. Skin looks brighter, clearer. Inflammation caused by too much sugar subsides. Weight loss is highly probable depending on how sugar-rich your previous diet was.
All in all, the better you start to look and feel physically, mentally and emotionally—the stronger the realization of the damage sugar wreaks on our mind, skin, and body will be.

5. Sweet Treats!

You'll find a handful of sugar-free alternatives for those times when you really want something sweet—and not a piece of fruit. Hint . . . there's a sugar-free, gluten-free cheesecake recipe that is to die for! These should be enjoyed sparingly, because although they're sugar-free, they're still caloric snacks. We wanna keep it in check, right? ;-)

What to Expect:

Weeks 1 and 2 are the most challenging because the body will (essentially) throw a temper tantrum. You may feel cranky, irritable and have hard cravings for sugar. The body wants its sugar fix!! Know that this is normal, and a part of the cleansing process. It *will* get easier. You're a warrior—stick it through.

Starting around Week 3, you should start to notice:

✓ **Greater mental clarity**

✓ **Some Weight-Loss**

✓ **Clearer, brighter skin**

✓ **Happier, more stable moods**

✓ **Foods may start tasting different as taste buds acclimate to cleaner foods. Sweet foods will seem "overly sweet."**

Overall, you should feel lighter, leaner, brighter and happier.

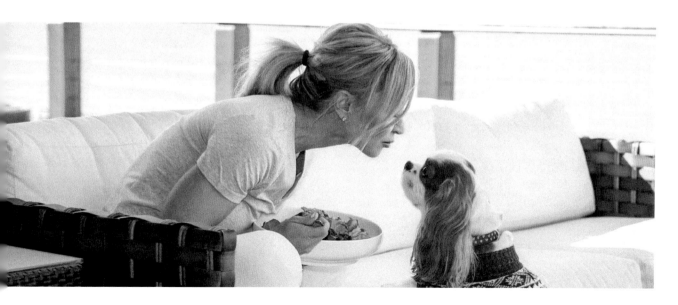

How to Work the Program

I t's easy and user-friendly! For the next 28-days, we're going to eliminate all added-sugars from your diet, in order to cleanse your mind and body of Sugar's negative effects and addictive qualities. It's a positive way to . . . *Reboot Your Life!*

After the 28-day Cleansing period, it will be up to you to decide whether to continue a NO-Sugar lifestyle or a LOW-Sugar Lifestyle *(under 24-grams per day for women, 36-grams for men)*. It's your body, your life—and your call.

Meal Selections

You'll find an array of recipes and ideas for No-Sugar Breakfasts, Lunches/Dinners, Snacks and Sweet Treats to choose from. Each day, simply:

- ✓ **Choose any Breakfast**
- ✓ **Choose any Lunch**
- ✓ **Choose any Dinner**
- ✓ **Choose any 1–2 Snacks**

You'll notice that I combined Lunch & Dinner recipes. I did this because lunch and dinner meals are really quite interchangeable nowadays. Some people prefer a heartier lunch and lighter dinner, others the reverse. So, it's really up to you. Choose what sounds best!

"Bulk" Recipes–Time Saver!

Some of the recipes, like the Quinoa Goat-Cheese Egg Muffins and the Bulgar Berry-Bake are made in "bulk," so that you can have several servings for the week. I'm all about making life easier! There's really no need to knock yourself out trying to cook several recipes every day.

Double the recipes that you like for the next day's breakfast, lunch and/or dinner. I do it all the time. It saves time and helps me stick to healthy eating vs grabbing something unhealthy because of a time crunch.

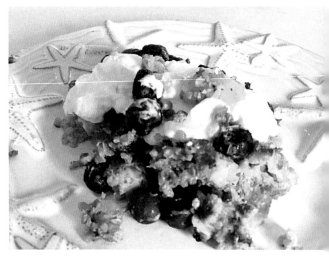

Warm Berry Blugar Bake

ANNIE PARKER CONFIDENTIAL

Live life beautifully ❀ by Shelli Pelly

What to Drink

Keep it pure & simple

✓ **Water**

✓ **Tea or Coffee, no sweetener**

✓ **Sparkling Water, squeeze of citrus optional**

✓ **Cappuccino or Latte, plain with favorite unsweetened nut-milk**

Alcohol

None, during the 28-day Cleanse. I know . . . You're a warrior, you can do this for 28-days. I guarantee.

Sugar-Free Sweeteners

Sugar-free doesn't have to mean bland and plain. Fortunately—there are some really great plant-based sweeteners that *do not spike your blood sugar, nor do they seem to have any of the negative effects of sugar.*

Swap them into recipes where you'd normally use sugar. In most cases, you won't know the difference. They're usually available in most grocery stores, but being a convenience freak—I order everything from Amazon and they're on my doorstep the next day or so ;-) Caveat—don't go crazy on sugar-free sweeteners . . .

Use Sugar-Free Sweeteners Sparingly–here's why:

The main argument against the use of sugar-free sweeteners, is the thought that eating sweet-tasting food and drink may encourage cravings for more sweetness. Sugar-free sweeteners some say, act as a crutch and don't actually eliminate cravings. For this reason, be judicious with your frequency of enjoying "sweet-treats."

The second concern, is that using these sweeteners to make, for example, sugar-free muffins, cakes, cookies, desserts, etc. tends to promote snacking and *extra consumption of calories* when we aren't hungry. So, if that sugar-free cheesecake tastes amazing, we're going to eat it "just because" it tastes good, not because we're hungry. That part makes sense to me.

My take

If desired, use sugar-free sweeteners *sparingly and in moderation*—with the knowledge that "sugar-free" is *not* a license to inhale every sugar-free cake, cookie and muffin in site. Don't fill your cabinets with processed, "sugar-free" junk food. The focus is on healthy, wholesome eating without sugar. Treats with sweeteners are . . . treats!

"Sweet treats" like a sugar-free cookie or a dessert, are made sparingly and infrequently, chez Pelly. If it's a birthday or special occasion, I'll make a small sugar-free dessert knowing that it's a treat, yet feel good knowing that it isn't a full Sugar-bomb.

I never buy sugar-free baked goods because they're just full of processed ingredients and crappy chemicals that don't nourish your body. In short, be mindful and use sweeteners sparingly. Baked goods and treats are just that . . . treats!

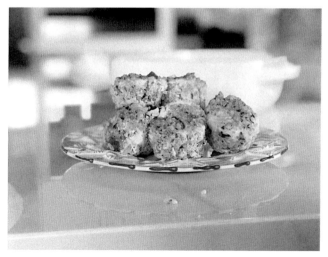

Quinoa Goat Cheese Egg Muffins

5 Tips for Success

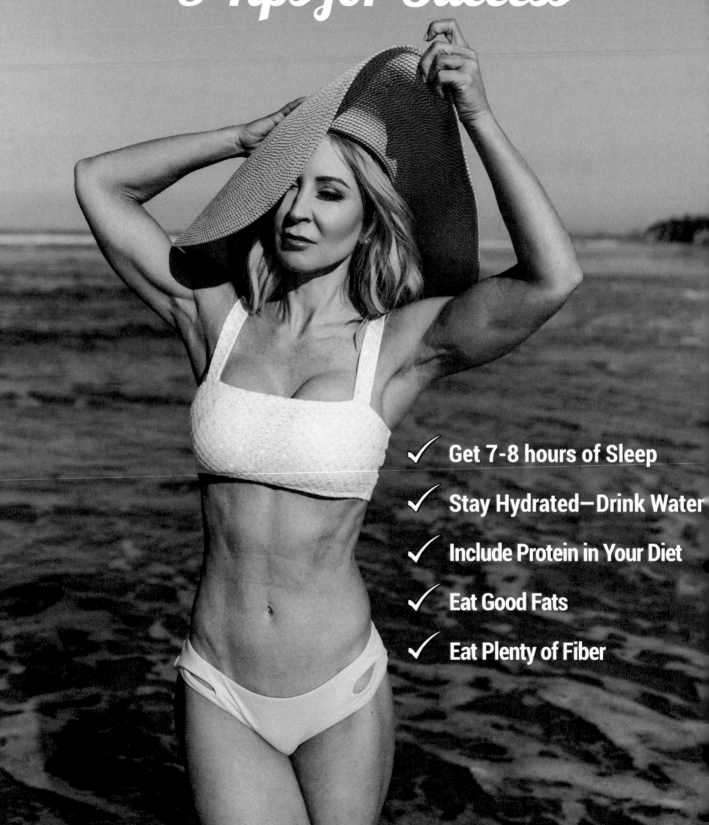

✓ Get 7-8 hours of Sleep

✓ Stay Hydrated—Drink Water

✓ Include Protein in Your Diet

✓ Eat Good Fats

✓ Eat Plenty of Fiber

5 Tips for Success

DO THESE 5 THINGS WITH THE PROGRAM

The key to a healthy lifestyle is setting yourself up for success. These 5 Lifestyle Habits serve as the *foundation* to help kick sugar from your life, for good. Pave the way towards vibrant energy, happy joyful moods, prettier more youthful skin, a healthier body and *your* most amazing life!

Here's what to do...

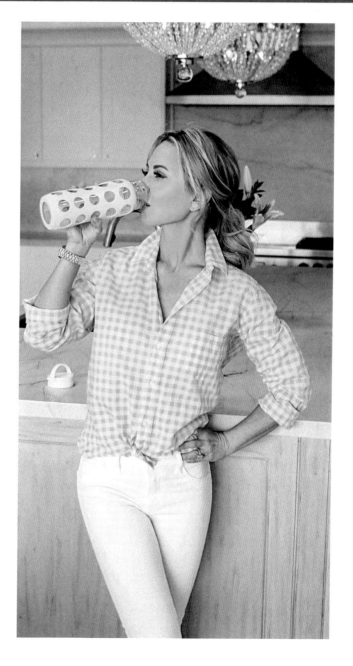

1. Get 7–8 hours of Sleep

Sleep helps curb sugar cravings! Getting 7–8 hours of quality sleep each night is not only incredibly important to our health it also helps to curb sugar cravings, *and* cravings for unhealthy foods which contribute to weight gain and obesity. Get your zzzzz's!

2. Stay Hydrated—Drink Water

I know—this sounds annoying. Why would we want *water* over a *cookie*?? Here's the thing: A lot of times when you crave something sweet —*your body is actually thirsty!* Drinking a big glass of water can take away that craving. More importantly—proactively staying hydrated goes a long way in stopping sugar cravings from starting in the first place. So . . . drink up, yo.

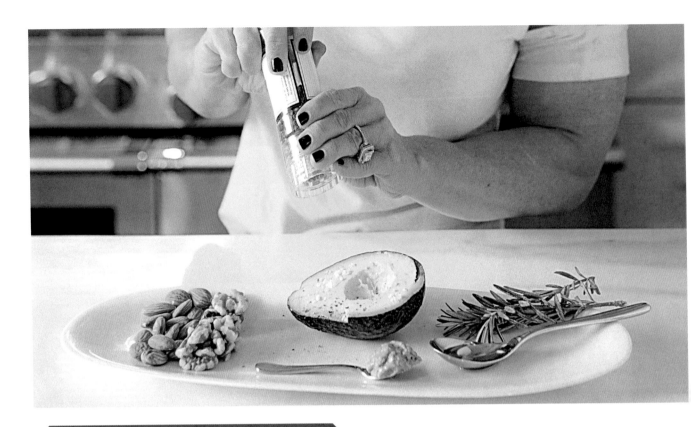

3. Include Plenty of Protein in Your Diet

There's a good reason for all of the lean proteins in our *28-Day Sugar Cleanse!* Proteins are a healthy way to feel fuller, longer and stabilize blood sugar. Plus, it will make the switch from a sugary-diet to no-sugar a much easier transition. Bonus—a high-protein diet is also important to building and defining muscles, so you'll see more benefit from your workouts!

4. Eat Good Fats

Good Fat in moderation does not make us fat. Too much refined sugar, carbs and processed foods make us fat. Our bodies *need* a certain amount of healthy fats like nuts, avocado, olive oil, salmon, etc., in order to function properly.

This is especially true when cleansing our bodies of a high-sugar diet and transitioning to a no or low-sugar diet. Here's why . . .

When burning energy, our body turns first to sugar. *When we eliminate sugar, the body starts burning its fat reserves.*

That's (partially) why you see all of those "Before and After Sugar" images of people looking chunky before kicking sugar—then super lean weeks or months later. Kicking sugar helps turn the body into a fat-burning machine.

Even better—once the body has gotten used to burning fat for fuel, *you'll start to crave healthy fats instead of sugar.* We like that!

5. Eat Plenty of Fiber

We're talking about high-fiber whole foods like kale, sweet potatoes, chia seeds, almonds, avocado, berries and whole grains like farro and quinoa. They all work to slow down the speed of digestion and stabilize blood sugar.

Fiber keeps us fuller, longer which is super helpful in curbing hunger and keeping us from reaching for something sweet and sugary!

What You'll Need

KEY PANTRY STAPLES USED IN THE RECIPES

For me, eating healthy and sugar-free as a lifestyle is all about making food *delicious, easy* and most importantly—*hassle-free*. To do this, I always keep the pantry full of Healthy (No-Sugar) Key Staples. All of the products below are items used in the Recipes, so set yourself up for success and stock-up!

All of the products are on Amazon, which means you can order online and have them delivered to your doorstep instead of futzing around the grocery aisles forever. Can you tell I'm an Amazon Prime fan? Lolol.

Pantry Staples

Quinoa

✓ **Healthy Grain**
✓ **Gluten-free, High Protein, High Fiber**

Quinoa is an ancient grain and one of today's most popular Superfoods. It is a much healthier substitute for white rice or pasta. I love its versatility and use it in soups, salads, stir-fry, breakfast bakes or as a porridge. Make a batch to have on-hand all week.

Bulgar Wheat

✓ **Whole Grain**
✓ **High Fiber, Iron, Manganese**

Bulgur is a whole grain with a similar texture and consistency to quinoa or couscous. Super versatile, use it in salads like Tabbouleh, stir-fry with veggies and chicken, in breakfast dishes like my Bulgar-Berry-Bake or as a porridge instead of oatmeal. Full of Fiber—it's satisfying and keeps you fuller, longer!

Chia Seeds

✓ **Essential Minerals & Antioxidants**
✓ **Fiber & Protein Rich**

Chia seeds are pretty much everywhere. A "superfood," they are the tiny black seeds from the Chia plant. We eat them *every day* Chez Pelly—no joke. Soak in alm ond milk with fresh berries for a healthy pudding (they expand & become gelatinous), add-in steel cut oats for Overnight Chia-Oat breakfast, sprinkle on salads, avocado toast or yogurt. Rich in fiber, omega-3 fatty acids and high-quality protein, you can't go wrong with these.

Ezekial Sprouted Bread

✓ **Rich in healthy nutrients & fiber**
✓ **No added sugar, no refined flours**

This is our go-to bread. Unlike most typical commercial breads which are are primarily made with refined or pulverized whole wheat and contain added-sugar, Ezekiel bread is made from organic, sprouted whole grains & legumes. Why Sprouted? Sprouting increases the number of healthy nutrients and reduces the number of antinutrients. Ezekial bread is not gluten-free, fyi.

Steel Cut Oats

Regular oatmeal is highly-processed, stripping out most nutrients. Steel-Cut Oats are minimally processed and therefore contain more fiber and density making them one of the healthiest grains you can eat. Soak overnight with fresh fruit for healthy breakfast, pulverize and use as "oat flour" in healthy oatmeal cookies!

Pancake & Waffle Mix

✓ **Sugar-free, Gluten-free**
✓ **High-fiber, Plant-based, Low-Carb**

A new find that I must share! Listen, there's a ton of sugar-free "junk food" on the market and believe me—I quickly pass on 99% of the products I vet. Which is why I was really excited to discover LAKANTO Pancake & Waffle Mix (available on Amazon). It's plant-based, high-fiber, no-sugar, gluten-free and most of all—it's really delicious. I like adding fruit to the mix, like ½ a chopped banana or fresh blueberries, which makes it extra moist. Best of all, you won't feel that yucky heavy feeling after eating these. If you like pancakes—try!

For Drinks

Orgain Organic Protein Powder

✓ **Smoothies & Oatmeal**
✓ **Helps repair muscles post-workout**

Protein powder is a super easy way to add more protein into your diet. Add a scoop into Smoothies, Smoothie-Bowls or Oatmeal for healthy, efficient protein to help you fill fuller, longer. Adding extra protein will also help to curb those sugar cravings! The Orgain Organic brand (available on Amazon) is the one I use. It's plant-based, sugar-free, organic, gluten-free, non-gmo, non-dairy *and* tastes pretty darn good. Of course use any Protein Powder that you like—just make sure it is sugar-free.

Matcha Green Tea Powder

✓ **Antioxidant-rich**
✓ **Boosts Metabolism, Enhances Mood**

"Matcha" is a type of green tea made by grinding young tea leaves into a bright green powder, which we then use a million different ways. Add it to: Smoothies, lattes, yogurt, baked goods or just as a hot cup of tea. It's got 137 times more antioxidants than regularly brewed *green tea!*

NutPods

✓ **Must try!**
✓ **Sugar-free, Dairy-free creamer**
✓ **Infused with amazing flavors**

NutPodz are a new find that I just have to share with you! It's not a Superfood, it doesn't have "amazing health benefits"—it's just a delicious, guilt-free way to add creaminess and decadent flavor to coffee, tea, oatmeal or smoothies! Oh—and they're shelf stable which means you can easily store in the pantry before opening.

Sugar-Free Sweeteners

Vanilla Monk-Fruit Liquid Sweetener

✓ **Like sweet vanilla-extract**
✓ **Zero-calorie, Zero-sugar**

I freaking love this stuff. It's like a hybrid of vanilla extract and liquid sweetener, but because it's made from Monk-fruit, it is sugar-free. Just 3–4 dashes are plenty to give a little sweetness to anything you like. I use it in my Chia Seed pudding, Overnight Oats or hot oatmeal.

Xylitol Plant-Based Sweetener

✓ **Use like granulated sugar in baking**
✓ **40% fewer calories than sugar**

Remember to use these no-sugar sweeteners sparingly. They key is to kick our cravings for sugar and sweetness. That being said, we all want to enjoy a little something sweet once in a while—so using plant based sweeteners is a really great option! I use Xylitol for my "family famous" No-Sugar Strawberry Cheesecake and 3-Ingredient Peanut Butter Cookies. They are da bomb! Straight 1:1 swap with regular sugar.

Erythritol Powdered Sweetener

✓ **Zero-calorie sweetener**
✓ **Use like powdered sugar**

Another great no-sugar sweetener, for sweet-treat recipes. I used this for the crust of my No-Sugar Strawberry Cheesecake and honestly it was sheer perfection. I *also* tested it for Buttercream Frosting and it was disgusting (weird aftertaste), so don't do that. It's much better in recipes where sugar isn't the star of the show.

Monk-Fruit "Maple Syrup"

✓ **Plant-based, Zero-sugar**
✓ **Use in recipes or over Pancakes**

I use the LAKANTO brand Maple Syrup. It smells and tastes exactly like real maple syrup, except it's not as thick. It's a touch thicker than water. I've used a Tablespoon in hot oatmeal with chopped pecans, or over blueberry protein pancakes and it's delicious! I *love* the satisfaction of eating pancakes and syrup *without* that disgusting, yucky, sugar-carb hangover. Instead you feel light & full-in-a-good-way.

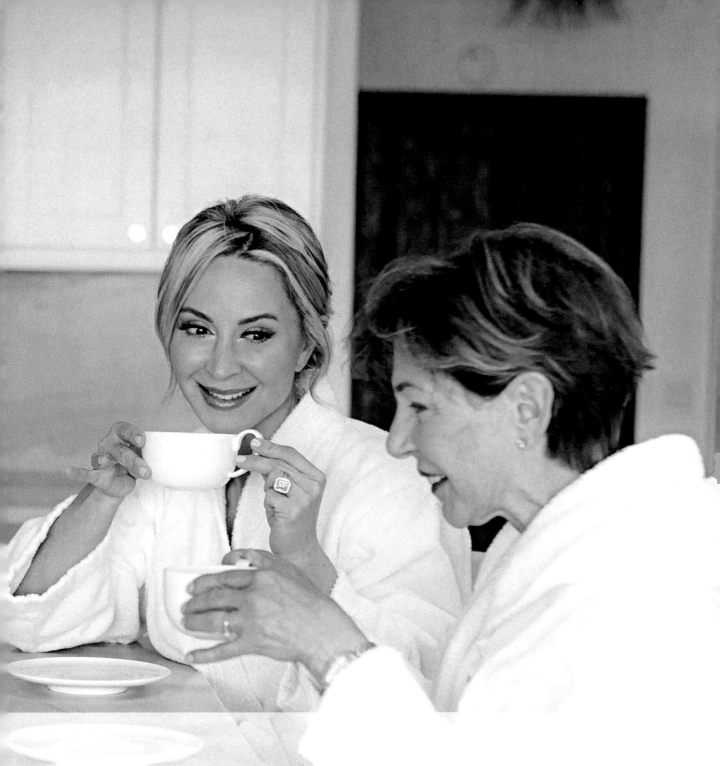

The Recipes

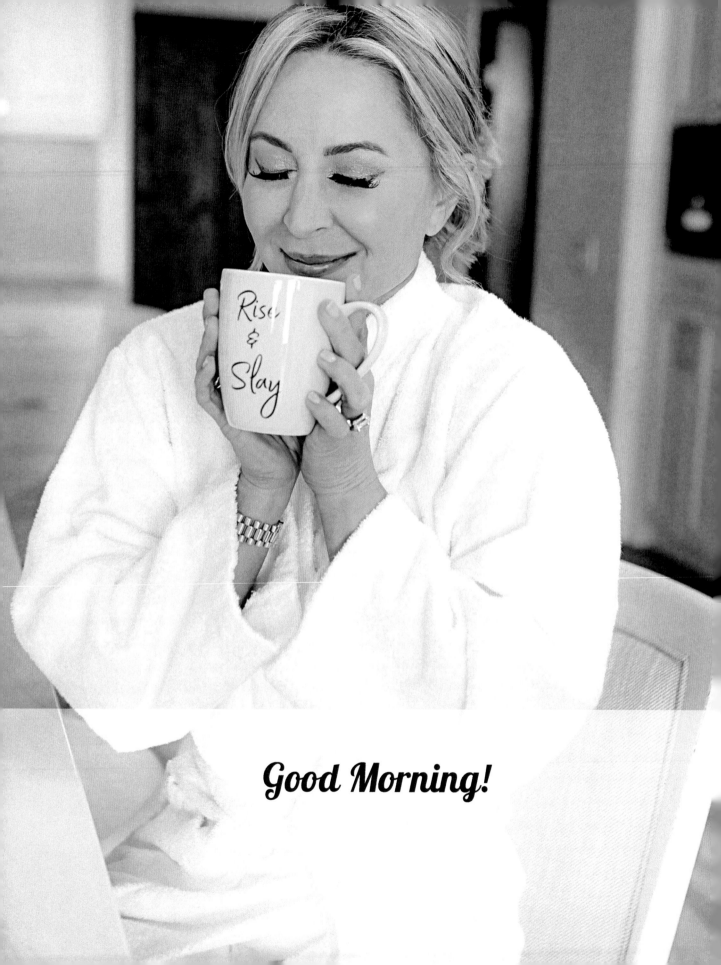

Good Morning!

Breakfast Ideas

SUGAR-FREE, HEALTHY & SATISFYING —SOME MAKE GREAT SNACKS TOO!

Greek Yogurt Berry-Coconut Bowl

+ ¾ cup plain Greek yogurt
+ 1 cup fresh mixed berries or ½ cup fresh pineapple chunks
+ 1 TB unsweetened shredded coconut
+ 4 roughly chopped macadamia nuts

Avocado Toast with Heirloom Tomatoes & Balsamic Drizzle

+ ½ mashed avocado on 1 piece Ezekial Bread (toasted)
+ sliced heirloom tomatoes
+ salt/pepper
+ fresh basil
+ drizzle balsamic vinegar

NOTE: Balsamic has sugar, but it is naturally occurring—not added.

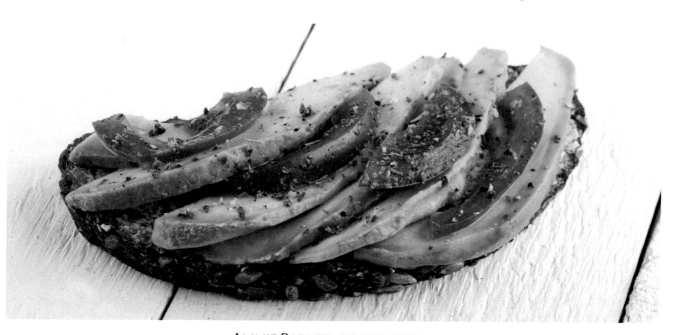

Oliver's Black Bean, Egg White & Veggie Breakfast Burrito

I ~~took~~ borrowed this creation from my husband, Oliver. It's one of my favorite breakfasts because it tastes and feels decadent. Plus it gets your day off to a great start with plenty of fresh raw veggies, egg whites for protein, and black beans for both protein *and* fiber. Yum!

+ 1 whole wheat tortilla
+ ⅓ cup shredded mozzarella
+ ⅓ cup black beans, drained
+ ½ cup liquid egg whites scrambled
+ 1 piece turkey bacon
+ ⅓ cup chopped spinach leaves
+ ¼ cup chopped mushrooms
+ 2 TB red bell pepper, chopped
+ chopped green onions

DIRECTIONS: Lightly toast both sides of tortilla in non-stick pan. Melt cheese on top. Remove from pan and assemble fillings: Beans, egg whites, turkey bacon, veggies. Roll & enjoy!

Overnight Pumpkin Oatmeal w/Diced Apple, Cinnamon & Walnuts

+ ⅔ cup steel cut oats
+ ¼ cup pumpkin puree (unsweetened, no additives)
+ ⅔ cup unsweetened almond milk
+ ½ tsp pumpkin pie spice or cinnamon
+ ½ tsp vanilla extract
+ 3–4 dashes of Vanilla Monk Fruit Liquid Sweetener (optional no-sugar sweetener)

DIRECTIONS: Combine all ingredients in a bowl and refrigerate overnight. In the morning, stir, top with chopped apple to taste, and 5 chopped walnuts. I love having this warm—just microwave 2-minutes and enjoy!

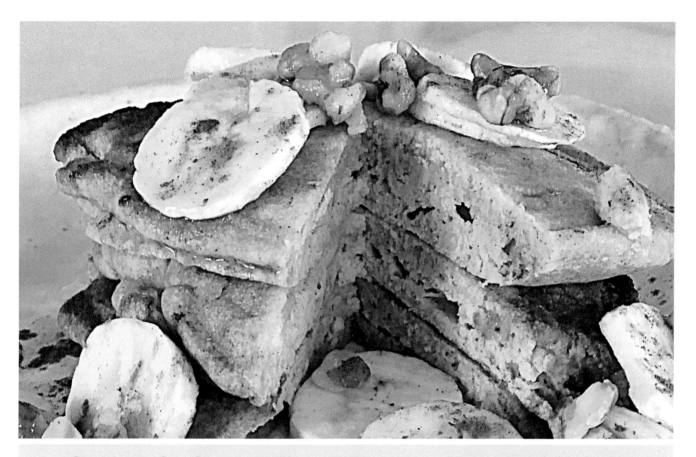

Pumpkin Pie Banana-Walnut Pancakes with "Maple syrup"

If you love pancakes, but not the schlumpy feeling that goes along with it, you *have* to try these! Made with *Lakanto Pancake & Waffle Mix: Plant-based, Low-Carb, No-Sugar, Keto, Gluten-Free & High Fibe*r, they're delicious, satisfying and leave you feeling, well . . . good! Oh, and the brands "maple syrup" made with Monk Fruit no-sugar sweetener puts this healthy pancake version over the top!

Make batter according to instructions, but add-in:

+ ½ tsp pumpkin pie spice
+ ½ tsp vanilla extract
+ ½ a banana, chopped into small chunks (makes 3–4 pancakes)

If batter seems overly thick, just add a little more water until it's the right consistency for pancakes. Cook over medium-heat in a non-stick frying pan sprayed with cooking spray.

TOP WITH: + ½ of banana sliced, + 5 chopped walnuts or pecans, + drizzle ⅓ cup Lakanto "Maple Syrup" flavored Monk Fruit, over the top—*optional*

Avocado Toast with Over-Easy Egg

+ 1 piece Ezekial Toast
+ ½ mashed avocado
+ salt & pepper
+ 1 fried egg, over-easy (place on top)

Overnight Blueberry-Almond Oats

+ ½ cup steel cut oats
+ 1 TB chia seeds
+ ¾ unsweetened almond milk
+ 3–4 dashes Vanilla Monkfruit Liquid Sweetener (optional)
+ ⅓ cup blueberries fresh or frozen
+ 1 TB slivered almonds

DIRECTIONS: Mix all ingredients in a bowl, except for almonds. Refrigerate overnight. In the morning, top with more fresh blueberries or strawberries if desired & slivered almonds.

HEALTHY SMOOTHIES

Breakfast, Snack, Post-Workout!

I love, love, love a delicious, healthy, efficient Smoothie—especially during Spring and Summer months when it starts getting warm out. Generally, you want to be super careful of bottled Smoothies or those that you buy at a Juice bar because honestly they can be loaded with added-sugars and tons of calories. Not so with these.

APC Very-Berry Fit & Glow Smoothie

Our Signature Breakfast Smoothie!

Our Signature Breakfast Smoothie for Spring & Summer is so berry-delicious, you won't believe it's healthy. Literally packed with antioxidants, 9-essential amino acids, Protein, key vitamins, fiber and good healthy fats, it's an incredibly efficient way to start your day.

+1 cup frozen blueberries
+ ½ large frozen banana
+ 1 TB almond butter, unsweetened
+ 3 TB hemp seed hearts
+ ½ scoop vanilla protein powder
(no added sugar)
+ ¾ cup vanilla almond milk,
unsweetened + ½ cup ice

Blend & Love it!

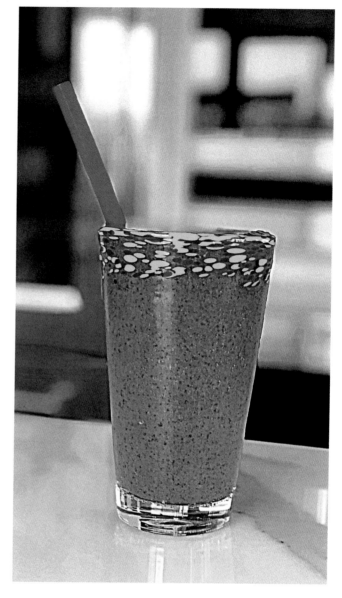

APC Very-Berry Fit & Glow
OUR SIGNATURE SMOOTHIE

Spinach Strawberry-Banana Protein Smoothie

+ generous handful of spinach leaves
+ ½ cup frozen strawberries
+ ½ frozen banana
+ 1-scoop vanilla protein powder
+ ¾ cup unsweetened almond milk
+ ½ cup ice

Blend

Oliver's Blueberry-Oat Protein Shake

+1 cup unsweetened vanilla almond milk
+ ½ frozen banana
+ 1 cup frozen blueberries
+ ⅓ cup steel cut oats
+ 1-scoop vanilla protein powder

Blend

Vanilla-Almond Matcha Smoothie

+ 1 banana, sliced & frozen
+ 1 TB powdered matcha
+ 1 cup unsweetened almond milk
+ ½ tsp vanilla extract OR 3 drops Liquid Vanilla Monk Fruit Extract (this is a non-sugar sweetener, optional)
+ ½ cup ice

Blend

Morning Espresso Protein Smoothie

+2 shots espresso or ¼ cup strong coffee
+ ½ cup unsweetened almond milk
+ ½ frozen banana
+ ½ tsp cinnamon
+ 1 scoop vanilla protein powder
+ ½ tsp vanilla extract OR 3–4 drops Liquid Vanilla Monk Fruit Extract (this is a non-sugar sweetener, optional)

Blend

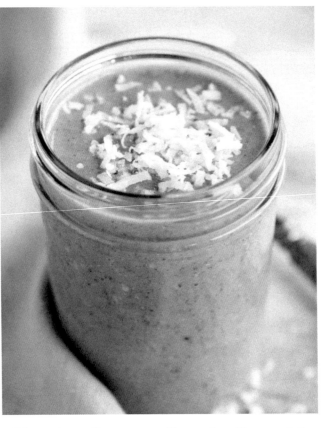

Morning Espresso Protein Smoothie

ANNIE PARKER CONFIDENTIAL
Live life beautifully ❀ by Shelli Pelly

Acai Protein-Smoothie Bowl

+1 frozen acai pack
+1 frozen banana
+ ½–¾ cup unsweetened nut-milk
+ ½ scoop vanilla protein powder

BLEND & pour into bowl. *Find Acai individually packed in the freezer section*

TOP WITH: ½ cup Blueberries, + ⅓ cup Sliced Strawberries, + 1 TB Unsweetened shredded coconut, + 7 Almonds roughly chopped.

MAKE-AHEADS FOR THE WEEK

I'm a fan of whipping up a few heat & eats that provide several servings for the week, and these dishes fit the bill. Healthy, filling, deelish and of course—no added sugars. Wink.

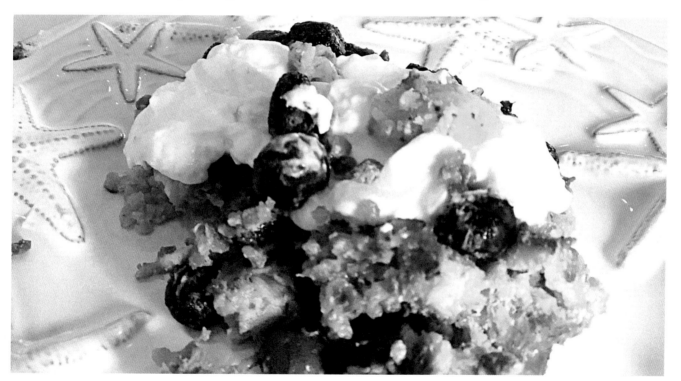

Warm Blueberry Bake with Bulgar Wheat

Warm Blueberry Bake with Bulgar-Wheat

+ ¾ cup bulgar wheat, uncooked
+ ½ cup steel cut oats, uncooked
+ 2 bananas, sliced
+ 3 cups blueberries, fresh or frozen
+ 2 ¼ cups unsweetened, vanilla almond milk
+ 2 eggs
+ 2 TB Monkfruit "Maple Syrup"
+ 1 tsp vanilla extract
+ ½ tsp cinnamon
+ ¼ tsp salt

Preheat oven to 375 degrees. Spray an 8 x 8 baking dish with cooking spray.

1. In a medium mixing bowl whisk together the almond milk, eggs, vanilla extract, "maple syrup", cinnamon and salt. Set it aside.

2. In the baking dish, evenly layer 1 of the sliced bananas over the bottom, then sprinkle half of the blueberries over the bananas.

3. Next, evenly spread the Bulgar Wheat & steel cuts oats all over the berries & banana.

4. Top with the 2nd sliced banana, and remaining blueberries

5. Slowly pour the liquid mixture evenly all over the ingredients.

6. Bake uncovered for 60 minutes.

7. Remove and let it cool.

8. Can be enjoyed warm or cold

9. Store in an airtight container and have breakfast for the week!

ANNIE PARKER CONFIDENTIAL
Live life beautifully ❁ by Shelli Pelly

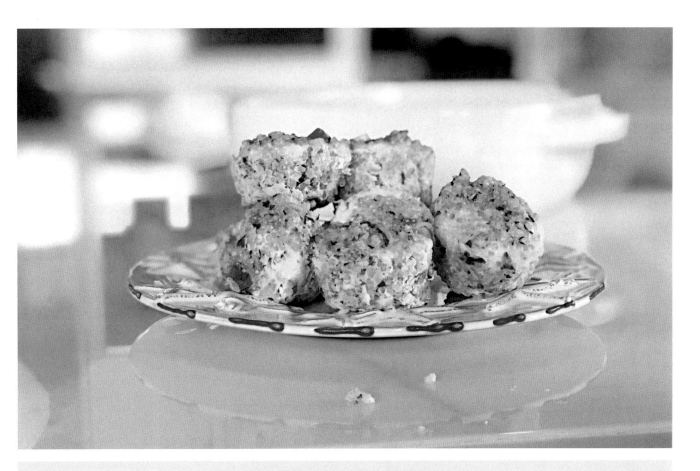

Veggie Quinoa Muffins

+ 2 cups quinoa, cooked
+ 3 whole eggs
+ ¼ cup liquid egg whites
+ salt & pepper
+ 4 oz herbed goat cheese or sundried tomato goat cheese, crumbled
+ 1 medium zucchini, grated
+ 4 TB chopped parsley
+ 1 ½ green onions, sliced thin

Preheat oven to 350 degrees. Combine all ingredients in a large bowl and mix to combine. Spray a 24-hole mini-muffin tin with non-stick spray and spoon mixture to the top of each cup. Bake for 15–20 minutes, cool for 10 minutes then remove from muffin tins & enjoy!

Mediterranean Quinoa Muffins

+ 2 cups quinoa, cooked
+ 3 eggs
+ ¼ cup liquid egg whites
+ salt & pepper
+ ½ cup crumbled feta
+ ½ cup julienned sundried tomatoes, drained
+ ½ cup sliced kalamata olives
+ ¼ cup fresh basil, juienned

Preheat oven to 350 degrees. Combine all ingredients in a large bowl and mix to combine. Spray a 24-hole mini-muffin tin with non-stick spray and spoon mixture to the top of each cup. Bake for 15–20 minutes, cool for 10 minutes then remove from muffin tins & enjoy!

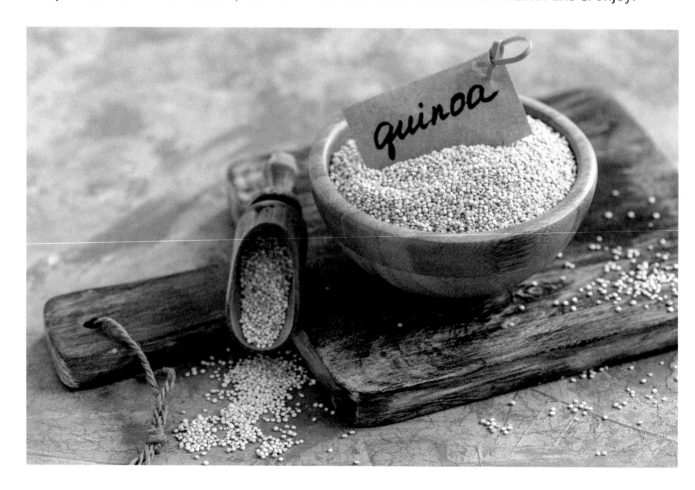

ANNIE PARKER CONFIDENTIAL
Live life beautifully ❀ by Shelli Pelly

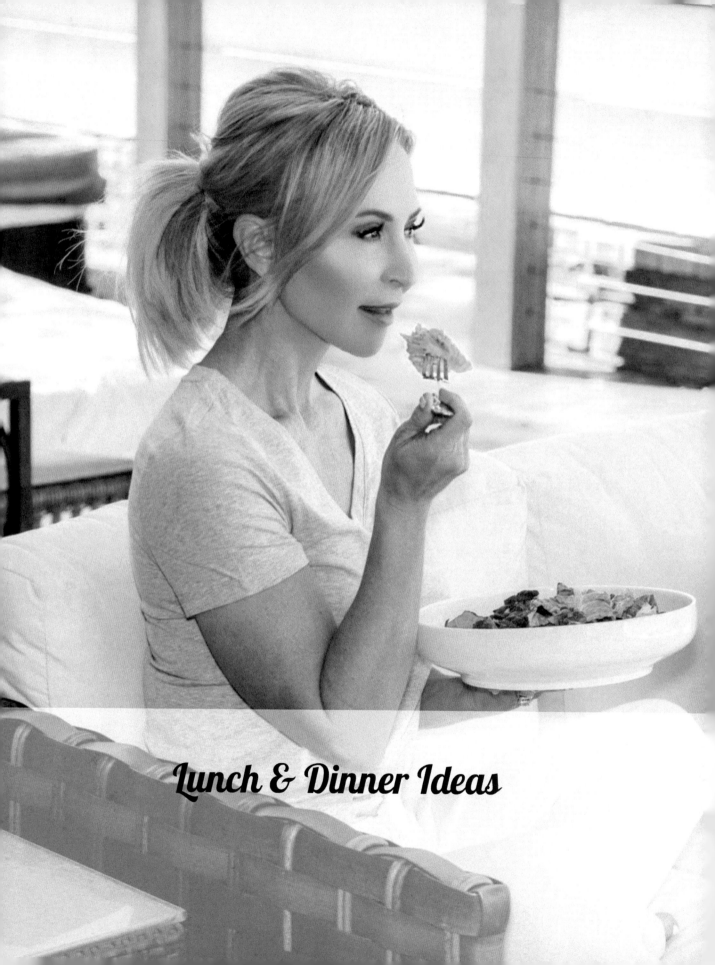

Lunch & Dinner Ideas

Lunch & Dinner Ideas

I decided to put lunch and dinner ideas together for a couple of reasons. First, to me lunch and dinner dishes are completely interchangeable and second—dictating what we "should eat" for lunch vs dinner is dated and confining. A great salad works just as well for dinner, whereas a fresh fish and veggie dish is equally satisfying for lunch.

In the end, just eat what sounds best to you. I think you'll love the selection and actually have fun mixing it up a bit. As always—these are all No-Added Sugar recipes.

SALADS AND BOWLS

Grilled Shrimp and Avocado Salad with Charred Pineapple

Serves 2

+ 1 ¼ pounds large shrimp, raw, peeled and deveined
+ 3 TB olive oil
+ kosher salt & pepper
+ 2 rings fresh pineapple, sliced ½-inch thick
+ 2 TB fresh lemon juice
+ ¼ small red onion, thinly sliced
+ ⅓ English cucumber, sliced into half-moons
+ 2 handfuls of watercress
+ ½ avocado, cut into chunks

1. Heat a grill pan over medium-high heat.

2. Toss shrimp with 1 TB of olive oil and sprinkle with a little salt and pepper. Brush pineapple with a little olive oil.

3. Grill pineapple on each side until it is slightly charred. Remove, cut into bite sized pieces and set aside.

4. Next, grill shrimp about 3 minutes each side or until pink. Remove and set aside.

5. In a medium bowl, whisk together lemon juice, 2 TB olive oil and salt & pepper. Add red onion and toss. Add in grilled pineapple, cucumber and shrimp. Toss together.

6. Fold in watercress and avocado—divide equally between 2 plates and enjoy!

Grecian-Style Shrimp & Farro Bowl

Serves 2

We always keep a sealed container of pre-cooked farro in the fridge, for convenience. It makes pulling together a healthy lunch or dinner like this one, super easy! Farro is an ancient grain, high in fiber and protein, that looks very similar to "fat" brown rice. I make it in our rice maker on the "brown rice" setting.

Make farro according to package instructions or remove from fridge if you've pre-made it!

For the shrimp: Grill or pan-fry 12-oz of fresh shrimp, peeled, deveined with tails removed. OR—use pre-cooked, frozen shrimp, defrosted (obviously). Cut into bite-sized pieces, place in a bowl and set aside.

For the dressing: In a small bowl, whisk together juice of 1 lemon + 1 clove garlic, minced + 1 tsp dried oregano + 2 TB olive oil + 1 tsp dijon mustard + salt-pepper to taste. Drizzle a little of the dressing over the shrimp & toss.

Chop veggies & assemble: 1-½ cups of diced English cucumber (no need to remove skin) + 1 cup cherry tomatoes, halved.

Assemble: In each bowl place ½–¾ cup of farro, half of the shrimp, cucumber & tomato. Drizzle dressing over each & toss. Sprinkle with 1–2 TB of crumbled feta. Enjoy!

Grilled Chicken & Avocado Salad with Apple Cider Vinaigrette

Serves 2

+ 2 boneless, skinless chicken breasts (about 6 oz each)

For the *Apple Cider Vinaigrette

*Makes 6–8 servings, so either cut recipe in half or just save extra vinaigrette in the fridge for a salad during the week

+ ⅓ cup extra virgin olive oil
+ ¼ cup apple cider vinegar
+ 1 TB dijon mustard
+ 1 TB monk fruit "maple syrup"
+ 1 TB Herbs de Provence
+ 1 garlic clove, minced
+ ½ teaspoon sea salt
+ ½ teaspoon fresh ground black pepper

For the avocado salad

+ 4 cups spinach or mixed greens
+ 1 cup cherry tomatoes, halved
+ ½ small red onion, chopped

+ 1 avocado, chopped into 1" cubes
+ 1 TB olive oil
+ 1 TB fresh cilantro, chopped
+ 2 TB grated Parmesan cheese
+ sea salt & fresh ground pepper to taste

Make the vinaigrette: In a small bowl, whisk together all of the Vinaigrette ingredients. Set aside.

Make the chicken: Rub with a little olive oil, then Season both sides with salt & pepper.

Cook on medium-low heat in a non-stick skillet until cooked through. This should take about 15 minutes, depending on the thickness. Let it rest as you make the salad.

For the Salad:

In a medium mixing bowl, add the greens, tomatoes, cilantro, cubed avocado and red onion. Drizzle ¼ cup of the Apple Cider Vinaigrette over the top, add in the Parmesan & toss everything together.

Divide the salad equally onto 2 plates. Slice the chicken breasts on the diagonal, and place one on top of each salad. Drizzle a teaspoon of vinaigrette over the chicken if you like. Enjoy!

Marinated Steak Salad with Cilantro-Lime Vinaigrette

Serves 2

+ (2) 6-oz flank steaks

For the steak marinade:

Optional! If pressed for time—skip it. Just season steak with salt, pepper and cook. Drizzle a little of the dressing over the steak right before serving. Just as good!

+ 4 TB lime juice, fresh squeezed
+ 4 TB extra-virgin olive oil
+ 2 TB sesame oil
+ 2 TB fresh cilantro, roughly chopped
+ 2 garlic clove, crushed

For the salad:

+ 6 cups of your favorite mixed greens
+ 1 small red bell pepper, julienned
+ ½ cucumber, sliced
+ 1–2 carrots, grated
+ ⅓ cup fresh cilantro leaves
+ 16 roasted, salted peanuts
+ ½ avocado, sliced for garnishing on top

For the salad dressing:

+ 2 TB extra virgin olive oil
+ 2 tsp sesame oil
+ 4 tsp lime juice, fresh squeezed
+ Pinch of salt & pepper

1. Add the marinade ingredients to a ziploc bag & swish them around to combine. Then add your steak, seal and marinate for at least 30 minutes.

2. Next, in a medium mixing bowl, toss all of your salad ingredients together except for the avocado—that will be used to garnish on top.

3. Whisk together the salad dressing ingredients, then pour over the salad mixture.

4. Toss and place salad onto a large plate.

Cook the steak:

5. Spray a small non-stick pan with cooking spray. Heat over medium-high heat.

6. Remove steak from the ziploc and pat lightly with a paper towel so it isn't dripping wet.

7. Season each side with salt and fresh ground pepper, then fry each side 3–4 minutes each (for medium rare).

8. Be sure to let the steak rest for ten minutes, otherwise the juices will run out & leave steak dry.

9. Slice against the grain into ¼" slices, then lay on top of the salad greens. slice against the grain and add to the salad. Garnish with the sliced avocado.+ 3 whole eggs + ½ cup liquid egg whites

Kale, Chicken & Spinach Salad w/Fresh Lime & Cilantro

Serves 1

In a medium mixing bowl, combine:

+ 1 chopped boneless, skinless chicken breast
+ 1 ½ cups of baby kale
1 ½ cups baby spinach
+ 1 medium carrot, shredded
+ 1 TB roasted sunflower seeds
+ ¼ avocado, sliced.

Make the dressing: In a separate bowl whisk together 1 TB extra virgin olive oil + juice of ½ lime + salt and pepper to taste. Add-in 2 TB chopped cilantro. Drizzle over salad & love your healthy meal!

Cherry Tomato, Goat Cheese & Arugula Frittata

Serves 4–6

Who says frittatas are a breakfast dish? They're just as perfect for brunch, lunch or even a light dinner, served with a fresh green salad. Serve hot or room temperature. Store leftovers in an airtight container, then simply heat for an easy next-day meal. Don't be intimidated—frittatas are super easy to make!

Just saute some veggies, make the egg mixture, pour over sautéed veggies & bake. Seriously—it's easy. I made this one with half whole eggs and half egg-whites. 100% egg white frittatas are a little too tough, IMO—so I like to mix in a few whole eggs for more tenderness. Awww!

+ ½ tsp kosher salt, ¼ tsp fresh ground pepper
+ 1 cup arugula, roughly chopped (baby spinach works also)
+ 1.5–2 cups cherry tomatoes, halved
+ 4-oz herbed goat cheese, crumbled
+ 2 TB parsley, finely chopped
+ ½ small yellow onion, diced
+ 1 TB extra virgin olive oil

1. Heat oven to 350-degrees

2. Heat an 8 or 9" non-stick frying pan over medium-high heat

3. In a large mixing bowl, lightly whisk the eggs together. Add in arugula, tomatoes, parsley, salt, pepper and crumbled goat cheese. Set aside.

4. Add olive oil to frying pan. Add onions and sautee until soft and translucent (2–3 min)

5. Remove from heat, add the egg mixture over the onions—moving ingredients around so they're evenly distributed.

6. Pop in the oven and bake about 30-minutes, or until it's browned and set in the middle. Let cool 10-minutes and enjoy! Serve with a fresh green salad if desired.

ANNIE PARKER CONFIDENTIAL
Live life beautifully 🌸 by Shelli Pelly

Salmon Over Farro & Arugula Salad with Dijon Vinaigrette

Serves 2

+ *(2) 4-oz salmon filets
+ **1.5 cups farro, cooked
+ ¼ cup lemon juice, fresh squeezed
+ 2 TB extra virgin olive oil
+ 2 TB dijon mustard

+ pinch of kosher salt
+ ½ small shallot, finely chopped
+ 1.5 cups cherry tomatoes, halved
3 cups arugula

* Omit the salmon if you're in the mood for a lighter dish. It's just as delicious!

** Farro is an ancient grain with a nutty flavor, chewy texture and appearance similar to brown rice. It is packed with protein and fiber (about 7 and 5 grams respectively, per ½ cup cooked)! We always have a Tupperware of it in the fridge, for an easy side. If you have a rice cooker—put it on the "brown rice" setting for perfect farro!

For the salmon filets: Heat oven to 400-degrees. Place tin foil on a baking sheet, lightly salt and pepper the fillets, place on baking sheet and bake for about 15-minutes or until opaque in the middle. Set aside.

In a large mixing bowl, whisk together the lemon juice, olive oil, dijon, shallot and pinch of salt. Add cooked farro and tomatoes, stirring to combine. Fold in arugula.

Divide farro salad mixture evenly between 2 plates, top each plate with a salmon fillet. Love it!

Salmon Quinoa Bowl w/Greens

Serves 2

Delicious hot or cold—save the other serving for lunch tomorrow!

+ (2) 4–6 oz fresh salmon filets, center cut (this is the best cut). Get the best quality possible, as the salmon is the star of this dish! Salmon is super rich, so I find that 4–6 oz is plenty for me. Oliver calls it a "Ladies portion."

If you're a grill master, or married to one, you can for sure grill your salmon. Personally, I hit the "Easy" button and bake it in the oven. Super easy & it's delicious.

Salmon:

Heat oven to 400 degrees.

Place tin foil onto a baking sheet and salmon filets on top.

Season with salt and pepper.

Bake for about 15–18-minutes. It should be opaque in the center.

Remove and let rest as you prepare the rest.

Balsamic Vinaigrette

+ 1 TB good quality balsamic vinegar
+ 1 ½ TB extra-virgin olive oil
+ ¾ teaspoon, dijon mustard
+ 1 garlic clove, minced

Quinoa Salad

+ 1 cup cooked quinoa, chilled
+ 2 cups arugula
+ ½ cup red onion, chopped
+ ¾ cup cherry tomatoes, halved
+ salt + pepper to taste
+ 1 tablespoons olive oil

Make the balsamic vinaigrette: Whisk together the balsamic vinegar, olive oil, dijon, garlic and salt and pepper. Set it aside.

Next, in a large mixing bowl, add the cooled quinoa, arugula, onion, cherry tomatoes and balsamic vinaigrette. Season with a little salt and pepper, then toss together.

Divide evenly between 2 bowls. Remove the skin from the salmon and top each salad with a salmon filet. Enjoy this healthy & filling meal!

Vegetarian Mediterranean Hummus Bowl

Serves 1

No cooking involved! Just assemble and enjoy for perfect lunch or light dinner! Note that you can always make your own hummus, but I prefer to buy mine for convenience. Whole Foods Original Hummus is one that I like.

In the center of a shallow bowl, place 1/3 cup of hummus, then surround it with these goodies:

+ ¾ cup cherry tomatoes, halved
+ 6–8 whole kalamata olives, pitted
+ handful of arugula or mixed greens
+ ¼ cup cubed feta
+ ½ cup chickpeas, drained and patted dry

Sprinkle everything with a pinch of sea salt, fresh ground pepper and ¼ tsp of dried oregano. Be sure to lightly rub the oregano between your fingers before sprinkling. This releases the flavor. Finally, drizzle with 1 TB of good quality olive oil and a squeeze of fresh lemon!

Black Bean & Tilapia Burrito Bowl

Serves 2

Fresh, easy, deliciousness in a bowl—without the tortilla! Just grill or "fry" the fish, assemble ingredients into a bowl and enjoy a healthy, yummy lunch or dinner. Use any flakey white fish, or swap out for chicken, grilled shrimp, or thinly sliced steak. It's all good!

+ 2 filets of tilapia or other white flakey fish, 6–8 oz each

+ (1) 15-oz can black beans, undrained
+ ¼ cup red bell pepper, chopped
+ ½ tsp ground cumin
+ ½ tsp garlic powder
+ salt & pepper to taste
+ 1 TB cilantro, chopped

+ 1 medium avocado, cut into chunks
+ 2 cups red cabbage, sliced thinly
+ ⅔ cup fresh tomato salsa
+ ½ cup cotija cheese
+ 1 lime, cut into wedges

1. Season both sides of the tilapia with a little salt, pepper, ground cumin & garlic powder.

2. Heat a medium non-stick frying pan over medium to medium-high heat. Add 1 TB olive oil. Fry fish covered for about 3-min each side, depending on thickness. Covering will keep some of the moistness in the fish. Remove and set aside on a plate.

3. In a small pot over medium heat, add the undrained can of black beans, ¼ tsp of ground cumin, ¼ tsp garlic powder. Bring to a simmer, add in cilantro and remove from heat.

Assemble: In 2 individual-sized bowls, divide ingredients equally and arrange alongside each other: Cabbage, beans, avocado, tomato salsa, tilapia (lightly broken into pieces). Sprinkle the cotija cheese over the top, garnish with fresh cilantro and lime wedge.

Asian Chicken Stir-fry with Broccoli & Light Peanut sauce

Serves 4

Light, healthy and packed with flavor, this dish is great for a couple days of healthy lunches or dinners. It's just protein packed chicken breasts, lots of veggies and just enough peanut sauce to add flavor & healthy fat.

+ 1-lb boneless, skinless chicken breasts, cut into 1" cubes
+ 1 TB sesame oil
+ 3 cups defrosted broccoli florets
+ 1 small red bell pepper, julienned
+ 1 8-oz can water chestnuts, sliced
+ 2 green onions, sliced thin
+ ⅓ cup roasted peanuts

Peanut sauce

+ ⅓ cup peanut butter, unsweetened, natural
+ 1.5 TB sesame oil
+ 2.5 TB rice vinegar
+ 2 TB low-sodium soy sauce or Tamari (gluten-free)
+ 1 TB water

Whisk together all ingredients for light peanut sauce and set aside.

Defrost the broccoli florets in the microwave, draining any excess water. Set aside with rest of prepared veggies (water chestnuts, red bell, green onions).

In a medium non-stick frying pan, heat the sesame oil. Add chicken cubes and fry until they are cooked through & no longer pink in the middle.

Add the red bell pepper plus 2 tablespoons of water and cook for another 2-minutes.

Reduce heat to low, add in broccoli, water chestnuts, green onions, peanuts and peanut sauce. Toss and allow everything to warm. Serve!

Southwestern Sheet-Pan Shrimp Fajitas-Fast!

Makes about 4 Fajitas

Use chicken breast instead of shrimp, if desired.

+ 1-lb large shrimp, fresh, peeled, deveined, tails removed
+ 1 small red bell pepper, julienned
+ 1 small orange or yellow bell pepper, julienned
+ ½ small red onion, sliced ¼" thick
+ 3 tsp chili powder
+ ¾ tsp ground cumin
+ ½ tsp cayenne pepper (or to taste)
+ 2 TB extra virgin olive oil
+ ½ tsp kosher salt + pepper to taste
+ 100% whole wheat tortillas

Garnishes

+ Sliced avocado
+ Fresh cilantro, roughly chopped (about 3 TB)
+ 1 lime, quartered

1. Heat oven to 400-degrees. Line a large baking sheet with tin foil.

2. In a large mixing bowl, toss together all ingredients up to and including the salt and pepper.

3. Spread mixture in a single layer on the baking sheet, bake on the middle rack for about 8–10 minutes or until shrimp are pink.

4. Remove shrimp from sheet & set aside in large mixing bowl.

5. Crank oven to "broil," and broil the veggies on the upper rack for about 4 minutes.

6. Remove and add to the shrimp. Toss together & assemble your Fajitas!

ASSEMBLE: Warm tortillas lightly in a pan. Fill with fajita mixture. Squeeze a little lime over the top. Layer ¼ of an avocado sliced, sprinkle with fresh cilantro. Enjoy!

Mediterranean Chicken or Shrimp Quesadilla

Serves 1—great use of leftover chicken

In a frying pan over medium heat, place:

+ 1 sprouted grain or 100% whole wheat tortilla
+ spread ¼ cup of hummus over entire tortilla.

On half of the tortilla layer:

+ ⅓ cup shredded chicken

+ ⅔ cup fresh spinach leaves
+ sliced roasted red bell pepper to taste
+ chopped kalamata olives to taste
+ 1 TB dried oregano
+ 2 TB crumbled feta.

Fold wrap in half, then cover pan to wilt the spinach (about a minute). Serve and enjoy!

Open-Faced Grilled Vegetable Sandwich with Goat Cheese

Serves 1

First, spritz a large grill pan over medium-high heat with cooking spray. Next, spray all veggies lightly and season lightly with salt, pepper & pinch of dried oregano.

Now grill them:

+ 1 portobello mushroom with stem removed and gills scraped out
+ 2 slices of eggplant about ½" thick
+ 4–6 slices of yellow squash.

Grill under tender, remove all veggies to cutting board to cool. Slice portobello into ½" slices.

Spread 2 tablespoons of herbed goat cheese (soft) onto 1-piece of toasted Ezekial Bread.

Now layer on:

+ roasted red bell pepper (I use jarred—way easier)
+ eggplant
+ portobello
+ yellow squash
+ 2–3 fresh basil leaves
+ sliced avocado

Enjoy!

Healthy Minestrone Soup

Serves 4–6

Perfect for busy weeks. Store in the fridge, for heat & eat lunches or dinners! Packed with fresh vitamin rich vegetables, beans for protein and farro which is a protein & fiber-packed whole grain, for a little staying power. You'll love it and feel amazing afterwards.

+ 3 TB, olive oil
+ 1 medium yellow onion, diced
+ 2 cloves garlic, minced
+ 3 large carrots, diced
+ 2 ribs celery, diced
+ (1) 14.5-oz can, crushed tomatoes
+ 1-lb of kale, thick stems removed and thinly sliced
+ 64-oz of vegetable broth
+ (1) 15-oz can kidney beans, rinsed and drained
+ 2 cups of prepared farro, cooked according to box instructions
+ ½ cup fresh basil, chopped, for garnish

In a large pot over medium-heat, heat olive oil then sauté onions and garlic together until soft (2-3 minutes).

Next, add in celery and carrots. Cook another 4-5 minutes until vegetables start to soften. Add in crushed tomatoes—continue to stir & cook for another 5–8 minutes.

Add in kale & vegetable broth (don't worry—the kale will cook down significantly). Bring everything to a simmer. Reduce heat to low, cover the soup, let it cook for 25-30 minutes.

Finally, add in the beans and farro. Let cook for anther 5 minutes. Taste the soup, and season with salt and pepper to taste.

That's it!

20-minute Chili, Light & Healthy

Serves 4

Chili is usually thought of as cold-weather food, but this particular recipe challenges that notion. It hits the perfect balance between light and filling. It won't leave you feeling heavy or sluggish— promise! Easy to make in 20-25 minutes, this is one of my favorite go-to recipes.

+ ½ small yellow onion, chopped
+ 1 small green bell pepper, chopped
+ 2 cloves garlic, minced—or squeeze of garlic paste
+ 1 TB olive oil
+ 1-lb ground chicken or extra-lean ground sirloin.
+ (1) 15-oz can Kidney Beans, drained
+ (1) 15-oz can diced tomatoes, with juices
+ 1 TB chili powder
+ 1.5 tsp dried oregano
+ red pepper flakes to taste

Garnishes

+ shredded cheddar to garnish (optional)
+ green onions to garnish (optional)
+ dollop of plain Greek yogurt (optional)

1. In a large non-stick frying pan, or Dutch oven over medium heat, add 1 TB olive oil. Add in onion, green bell pepper and garlic. Sautee until the mixture is soft, about 2-minutes. Season with a little salt (just a pinch)

2. Raise heat to medium-high. Add in ground chicken or sirloin, season with a little salt, and cook until meat is browned. Add in kidney beans and diced tomatoes, stir to incorporate.

3. Add in chili powder, oregano and red pepper flakes. Turn heat down to medium, and stir for another minute or two, just to allow flavors to marry.

That's it! Garnish with a dollop of plain greek yogurt, a sprinkle of sliced green onions, and a little shredded cheddar (about 2 TB). Enjoy!

ANNIE PARKER CONFIDENTIAL
Live life beautifully ❀ by Shelli Pelly

Healthy Nibbles

Sugar-Free Snacks We Love!

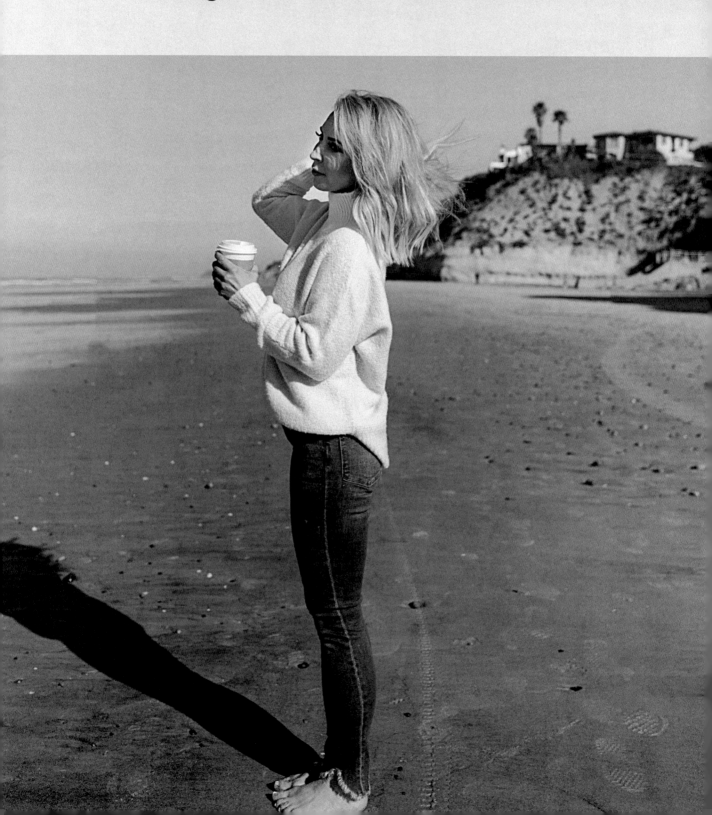

Healthy Nibbles

SUGAR-FREE SNACKS WE LOVE!

Healthy, no-added sugar, perfectly filling little snacky treats that taste as good as they make you feel!

1. ***Almond-Butter-Yogurt Spread:*** Mix together 1 TB unsweetened almond butter & 1 TB plain greek yogurt. Spread on apple wedges.

2. ***Berry Nutty Yogurt:*** Plain, unsweetened Greek yogurt + sliced berries + chopped pistachios

3. ***Cinnamon Sweet Potato:*** ½ baked sweet potato + 1/2 TB melted butter + sprinkle of cinnamon. Yum, right?!

4. ***Jimaca Fries:*** Cut 1–2 jimacas into slices like french fries. Toss with a little olive oil. Season with salt, pepper, garlic powder and turmeric. Bake at 400-degrees on a baking sheet for 20-minutes.

5. ***Crunchy Chickpeas:*** 1-can chickpeas rinsed and dried. Bake on baking sheet at 400-degrees for 20-minutes. Remove from oven. Sprinkle with sea salt & curry. 2-servings.

6. ***Avocado Toast & Cottage Cheese:*** Mash ½ avocado on toasted Ezekial or sprouted bread. Season with salt & pepper. Spread ¼ cup cottage cheese over the top. Enjoy!

7. ***Hummus & Red Bell Pepper Wedges:*** Red bell pepper wedges & ¼ cup Hummus.

8. ***Cherry tomatoes + Mozzarella + Balsamic Bowl:*** In a small bowl, add 1-cup cherry tomatoes halved, 1-oz fresh mozzarella cubed, 2–3 fresh basil leaves torn, 1 TB balsamic vineger, salt & pepper.

9. ***Chia Seed Pudding w/Berries:*** (Make-ahead) In a bowl mix 3 TB chia seeds, ½ tsp vanilla extract, ½ cup unsweetened vanilla almond milk, mix. Let sit in fridge for an hour. Chia seeds will absorb milk and expand like tapioca pudding. Top with ½ cup blueberries & 4 chopped almonds. Add more milk if desired.

ANNIE PARKER CONFIDENTIAL
Live life beautifully ❧ by Shelli Pelly

Healthy Nibbles

SUGAR-FREE SNACKS WE LOVE!

10. *Hard Boiled Eggs:* Make ahead of time & store in fridge for easy grab-n-go snacks.

11. *Ricotta Cheese and Pears w/Cinnamon:* In a bowl combine: ½ cup low-fat ricotta cheese, 1 ripe pear diced, sprinkle with cinnamon & 4 chopped almonds.

12. *Tuna Bite Crackers:* Mix ½ can albacore tuna in water, with 1 tsp low-fat mayonnaise & 1 tsp dijon. Enjoy with multi-grain crackers, like CrunchMaster Multi-grain—no sugar, gluten-free, non-GMO & whole grain.

13. *Avocado Crackers:* ½ ripe avocado mashed. Slather on multi-grain crackers, sprinkle with sea salt & ground pepper. Add fresh heirloom tomato slices if desired.

14. *Toast w/Greek Yogurt & Mixed Berries:* 1-slice sprouted bread or Ezekial bread, toasted. Slather plain Greek yogurt or low-fat ricotta cheese, top with fresh sliced strawberries & blueberries.

15. *Tomato Avocado Melt:* 1-slice sprouted bread or Ezekial bread, toasted. ½ avocado mashed onto toast, salt/pepper to season. Layer on 3–4 fresh sliced heirloom tomatoes, salt/pepper to season, top lightly with fresh mozzarella & melt under broiler.

16. *Strawberry-Banana Protein Smoothie:* 8–9 medium frozen strawberries, ½ frozen banana, 1 scoop vanilla protein powder, ½–¾ cup unsweetened vanilla almond milk. Blend & enjoy.

17. *Whole fruit:* Choose a fruit with a lower GI (Glycemic Index) such as: apples, oranges, pears. They're sweet, deliciously refreshing and best of all, portable so you can eat on the go, and keep them in your desk at the office.

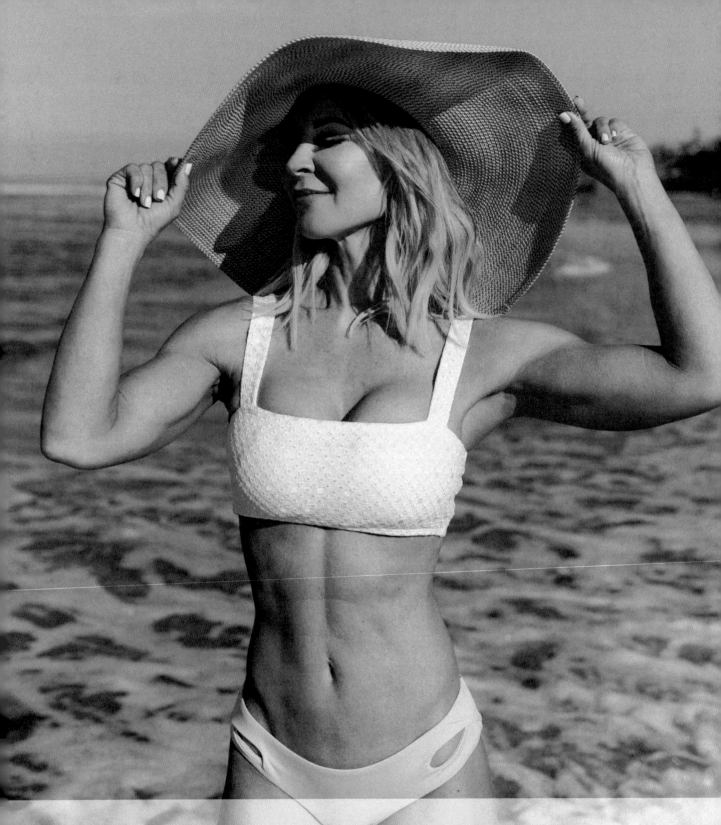

Sugar-Free Sweet Treats!

Sugar-Free Sweet Treats

3-ingredient Peanut Butter Cookies

Heat oven to 350-degrees.

Mix together:

+ 1 cup unsweetened natural peanut butter
+ ½ cup Xylitol (no-sugar sweetener)
+ 1 egg

Roll into balls and place on non-stick baking sheet. Use a fork to press balls flatter, making a criss-cross pattern. Bake 8–10 minutes and enjoy!

Peanut-Butter Maple & Cacao Energy Balls

In a mixing bowl add & mix together:

+ 1 cup peanut butter, unsweetened
+ ¼ cup flax seeds
+ 3 TB hemp seed hearts
+ ½ cup raw almonds, chopped
+ ¼ cup unsweetened coconut flakes
+ ⅓ cup Lakanto-brand no-sugar "Maple Syrup" (see Pantry List).

Mix to incorporate. Roll into 1-inch balls. Roll half of the batch through cacao powder (I use Hershey's dark 100% cacao powder), roll the other half through flax seed meal. Eat "as is" or freeze! Keep stored in an airtight container in either the freezer or fridge.

ChocZero Almond & Sea Salt Dark Chocolate Bark

The easiest sweet-treat of all . . . Just buy them on Amazon! I know, right?! Sweetened with Monk-Fruit, you will never know the difference. Dark chocolate, with chopped almond and sea salt for the perfect salty-sweet balance.

They come individually wrapped and are just perfect for those times when you just want "a little something sweet." These are always on hand in the Pelly household!! They come in a few varieties such as almond & sea salt, peanut & sea salt, and coconut. I've even unwrapped a few, broken into bite sized pieces and served in a pretty silver candy dish when friends have come over for a glass of red wine. And yes, I told them. ;-)

8-Ingredient Fresh Strawberry Cheesecake

I tested this recipe on the ultimate "I LOVE SUGAR" person. My Dad. I had already tested, tasted and loved it, but knowing that my palate had adapted to no-sugar, I needed to call in the big guns. If Dad loved it—I knew it was a winner.

I watched as he cautiously lifted a bite to his mouth and began carefully chewing, ready to spit it out at a moment's notice. Suddenly his eyebrows lifted in surprise—Is this sugar-free?" Yes. He loved it. So much so, he finished off the entire cheesecake in a matter of days, Lolol.

Alarmingly easy to make and only 8-ingredients. Perfect for a special occasion. Place on an elegant cake stand, and arrange fresh-sliced strawberries on top for a chic-treat!

For the Crust

Heat oven to 350-degrees. In a medium mixing bowl combine:

+ 2 cups of almond flour
+ ⅓ cup butter, melted
+1 tsp vanilla extract
3 TB granulated Xylitol.

Mix together, then press into the bottom of a 9-inch spring-form pan that has been sprayed with cooking spray. Bake for about 10-minutes. Remove and let cool.

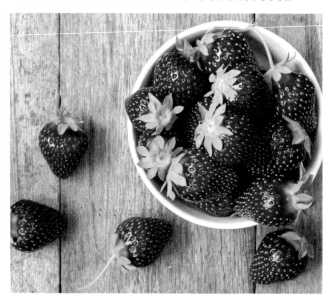

For the Cheesecake Filling

In a large mixing bowl, combine:

+ 32-oz (4 regular 8-oz packages) of room-temperature light cream cheese
+ 3 eggs
+ 1 ¼ cups of powdered Erythritol (don't use granulated—it'll give the cheesecake a really weird texture.)
+ 1 TB lemon juice, fresh squeezed
+ 1 tsp good quality vanilla extract.

First, on medium-speed, beat the cream cheese and Erythritol together until light and fluffy. Beat in the eggs one at a time. Finally, reduce speed to low and mix in lemon juice and vanilla extract. Pour into cooled Almond Flour crust, and bake for about 50-minutes or until the center is only slightly jiggly. You do want a little jiggle otherwise the cheesecake will be overbaked.

Remove from the oven and allow to completely cool in the pan, then place in the refrigerator 4–6 hours. Remove from Spring-form pan, top with fresh sliced strawberries and love it!

ANNIE PARKER CONFIDENTIAL
Live life beautifully ❁ by Shelli Pelly

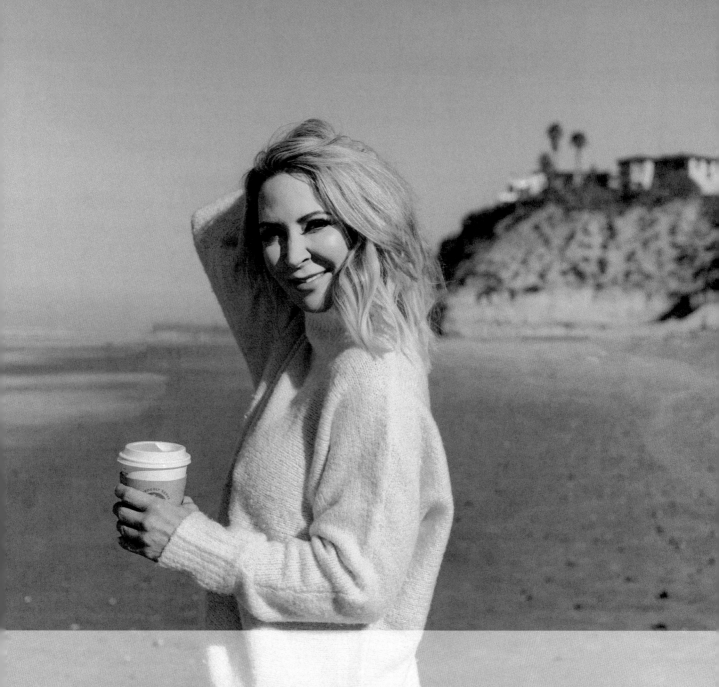

FAQ's

Frequently Asked Questions

1. Can I have fruit? Fruits have sugar, right?

You can have whole fruit but steer clear of fruit juices. In their natural state, whole fruit contains fiber, water and sugars that naturally occur within the fruit and thus are ok to eat in moderation. When eaten whole, fruit is a healthy option. However, fruit juices are not a healthy option, because the fiber has been separated out—leaving you with a glassful of "sugar," that will cause the insulin surge we want to avoid.

2. What about Honey, Maple syrup, Molasses or Agave Syrup/Nectar? I see healthy recipes using these all the time.

In short, these items are just a different form of sugar, so on this Program, they're a "No." When I have eaten honey, thinking it was a healthier option—I'd get a raging, splitting headache. Exactly like a sugar rush. The body clearly saying—"I don't care if it's honey, honey—me no likey."

3. What sweeteners (sugar alternatives) are used in the Program?

Part of the reason that I've found going sugar-free fairly "easy," is the existence of some pretty damn good non-artificial sugar alternatives that can easily be swapped into your favorite recipes so it doesn't feel like you're being deprived.

Excellent alternatives include:

✓ Stevia
✓ Monk fruit extract
✓ and sugar alcohols like Xylitol and Erythritol

You'll still want to watch your intake—but it's really nice to enjoy a cookie or muffin every once in a while.

There are 3 sugar substitutes that I love and use in my own life. They are:

1. **XYLITOL:** Xylitol is a sugar alcohol that comes from natural sources like birch trees, and has about 40% fewer calories than sugar. Since the body absorbs it at a slower rate than it absorbs sugar, it doesn't cause the same dramatic spikes in our blood sugar. Baking with it is super easy. It's a 1:1 swap, used just like sugar.

2. **ERYTHRITOL:** Erythritol is also a sugar alcohol that comes from natural sources like fruits, and it's used in sugar-free gum, candies, chocolates, etc. It comes in granulated and powdered versions—great for baking at home!

3. **MONK FRUIT EXTRACT:** Monk fruit has actually been used for centuries in Chinese medicine, receiving FDA approval in the U.S as a sweetener in 2010. It's natural, has zero calories and is anywhere from 100-250 times sweeter than sugar. It's also thought to have antioxidant properties.

Stevia is also fine to use, if you prefer.

4. What about sweeteners like Equal, Sweet 'n Low, Splenda or Sugar Twin?

So, there are some recent studies indicating that these particular sweeteners may actually correlate to the increase of obesity and diabetes. For these reasons, I chose to err on the side of caution, and did not include them in the Program.

5. What about everything in moderation? Can't I have a cookie, brownie or a piece of cake as a treat once in a while?

A qualified "Yes"—as long as they're made with an approved sugar substitute such as Xylitol, Erythritol or Monk-Fruit. All 3 are used regularly in sugar-free recipes and honestly, you'd never know the difference—they're that good. The only difference is a good one—the absence of that yucky sugar high / sugar crash and the negative effects of sugar on the body.

Sugar-in-moderation: I challenge you to shift your perspective a bit. Instead thinking of a "real-sugar" brownie or cookie as a treat in moderation, raise the bar. Your "moderation" treat is now a sugar-free brownie, cookie or dessert. Of course you know my mantra . . . "You're the boss of you." It's your body, your life and your decision—but given all of the delicious sugar-free options at our fingertips, there's no reason to fill your beautiful-self with toxicity.

6. After the Program, how much daily added-sugar is "ok" for me to have?

Under 24-grams per day, for women, 36-grams for men. This, according to the ADA (American Diabetes Association). Of course zero is always best, but I'm a realist—and no one eats perfectly all the time. Having this number in mind, will make you much more aware of what you're eating. Honestly, I suspect that you'll get so used to feeling good, that sugary processed foods won't be as enticing as they once were.

7. I have allergies or specific dietary needs. Can I still do the Program?

First and foremost, please consult a medical professional, before starting any new eating program. Safety first.

That being said, some of the recipe ideas in the Program may include gluten, nuts, shellfish, and dairy products. It isn't geared towards any one specific dietary program other than eliminating sugar and focusing on the use of whole and minimally processed foods.

ANNIE PARKER CONFIDENTIAL
Live life beautifully ❀ by Shelli Pelly

In Closing

In closing, I'd like for you to remember a few things that I've always found helpful throughout life: First and foremost—you're the boss of you, and the ultimate decision maker of the trajectory and direction of your life. Whether you go left or right, is totally your call.

The fact that you've read this book, says that you are someone who strives to learn, explore new ideas or concepts, then puts in the effort to grow and evolve. It tells me that even if you've been in a rut (and who hasn't?)—you're the one who will pull yourself up and forward.

The difficulty of creating a new habit, will lie in direct correlation to your starting point. For example, someone who eats a high-sugar diet, filled with lots of processed foods will have more of an initial challenge adapting to the Sugar Cleanse, than someone who eats relatively healthy but just wants to tighten it up.

That is OK! If you are the high-sugar person—know that it will be more of a challenge—then just keep going! On a positive note, the greater the change, the more impressive the results will be. The fact that you're making positive changes for yourself despite the challenge, is incredibly commendable. Total respect! Fist bump.

Be sure to visit me on the Blog—annieparkerconfidential.com, and of course as a Sugar Cleanse reader, you're invited to join our private Facebook Group where you can share and connect with me, and other women.

See ya on the blog!

Xoxo,

-Shelli

Made in the USA
Middletown, DE
18 September 2024

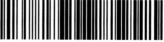